Running

The Things Men Will Never Tell You About the Sport

(The Ultimate No-fluff Guide to Running With Confidence as You Age)

William Watson

Published By **Darby Connor**

William Watson

All Rights Reserved

*Running: The Things Men Will Never Tell You
About the Sport (The Ultimate No-fluff Guide to
Running With Confidence as You Age)*

ISBN   978-1-7777356-8-5

Legal & Disclaimer

The information contained in this book is not designed to replace or take the place of any form of medicine or professional medical advice. The information in this book has been provided for educational & entertainment purposes only.

The information contained in this book has been compiled from sources deemed reliable, and it is accurate to the best of the Author's knowledge; however, the Author cannot guarantee its accuracy and validity and cannot be held liable for any errors or omissions. Changes are periodically made to this book. You must consult your doctor or get professional medical advice before using any of the suggested remedies, techniques, or information in this book.

Table Of Contents

Chapter 1: Marathon Training For Runners over Forty

Understanding the Unique Needs of Older Runners

As we age, our bodies go through diverse changes that may affect our walking overall performance and commonplace nicely-being. In this subchapter, we are able to discover the specific desires of older runners and provide treasured insights that will help you keep taking walks robust properly into your 40s, 50s, 60s, and past.

Running over forty calls for a greater focus on harm prevention and recuperation Our bodies take longer to heal as we age, and it's miles critical to contain right heat-up and funky-down physical games, stretching bodily video games, and circulate-schooling sports activities to hold flexibility and reduce the threat of injuries.

Marathon training for runners over forty calls for a extra slow and aware approach. It is crucial to listen for your frame, modify your education plan therefore, and prioritize healing to keep away from burnout and optimize your typical performance on race day.

When it involves on foot tools and tool for older runners, comfort and help come to be paramount. Invest in extraordinary taking walks footwear that provide ok cushioning and stability, and keep in mind the usage of compression socks or sleeves to decorate blood skip and decrease muscle ache.

Running for weight loss and body composition changes within the ones over forty may be difficult because of a slower metabolism. However, through the use of way of enforcing a nicely-balanced weight-reduction plan, incorporating electricity training carrying occasions, and retaining a consistent taking walks recurring, you may attain your weight loss desires and decorate body composition.

Running packages and sporting activities for novices over forty have to cognizance on progressively building patience and electricity. It is crucial initially shorter distances and lower intensity wearing activities, permitting your body to conform to the desires of walking at the identical time as minimizing the risk of overuse injuries.

Maintaining joint health is vital for older runners. Incorporating physical sports that improve the muscle companies surrounding your joints, which incorporates hips and knees, can assist alleviate pressure and reduce the risk of joint ache or degenerative conditions.

Running for intellectual and emotional well-being in people over 40 has severa blessings. Regular on foot can help lessen pressure, decorate temper, and increase self-self notion, important to increased standard nicely-being.

Running for cardiovascular fitness and ailment prevention in the ones over 40 is an extremely good way to beautify coronary coronary heart fitness and decrease the threat of continual illnesses along side coronary heart disease, diabetes, and hypertension. Engaging in normal aerobic workout, such as walking, facilitates help the coronary coronary coronary heart and beautify everyday cardiovascular health.

Running for increased strength and power in human beings over forty can assist combat age-related fatigue and growth normal electricity tiers. Regular on foot stimulates the manufacturing of endorphins, boosts metabolism, and enhances ordinary physical and intellectual stamina.

Lastly, course strolling and outdoor adventures provide an interesting and clean enjoy for runners over forty. Exploring nature, hard terrains, and breathtaking sceneries can invigorate your strolling ordinary and add a experience of adventure on your fitness adventure.

Understanding and addressing the specific wishes of older runners are critical for preserving a wholesome and amusing taking walks life-style. By enforcing the recommendation furnished in this subchapter, you can keep to excel in your walking endeavors and encompass the numerous bodily, intellectual, and emotional blessings that walking has to offer.

Training Plans and Strategies for Marathon Success

When it includes marathon education, right planning and technique are important, especially for older adults. As we age, our our our our bodies require extra care and interest to save you accidents and ensure vital performance. In this subchapter, we are able to discover schooling plans and strategies specially designed for runners over 40 to assist them benefit marathon fulfillment.

One crucial element of training is frequently building mileage and depth. Older adults won't get higher as rapid as extra youthful runners, so it's far essential initially a conservative approach. Begin with a base education phase, that specialize in increasing your weekly mileage grade by grade. Incorporate relaxation days and pass-training sports like yoga or swimming to promote restoration and prevent overuse accidents.

To decorate marathon fulfillment, it is crucial to encompass each prolonged runs and velocity wearing activities in your education plan. Long runs construct staying electricity and intellectual electricity, at the equal time as tempo exercise workouts enhance your walking efficiency and assist you maintain a faster tempo. However, older runners have to be cautious not to overdo it. Aim for one longer term in keeping with week, little by little growing the space, and contain one or pace physical games constant with week, which include durations or tempo runs.

In addition to mileage and intensity, strength schooling is crucial for older runners. It allows save you muscle imbalances, improves common body power, and decreases the hazard of accidents. Include sports activities that target the main muscle companies, collectively with squats, lunges, planks, and push-ups, as a minimum two instances in keeping with week.

Another crucial technique for marathon achievement is right vitamins and hydration. As we age, our our bodies may also furthermore require considered one in every of a kind nutrient ratios and higher fluid consumption. Focus on ingesting a balanced weight-reduction plan wealthy in lean proteins, whole grains, give up result, and veggies. Stay hydrated with the useful resource of eating enough water at some stage in the day, specially during schooling runs.

Lastly, keep in mind the significance of relaxation and restoration. Adequate sleep and relaxation days are essential in your frame to restore and adapt to the schooling stimulus. Incorporate stretching, foam rolling, and other healing techniques to save you muscle tightness and promote joint fitness.

By following those training plans and strategies, older adults can maximize their marathon fulfillment. Remember, marathon training is a adventure, and it is vital to concentrate to your frame, make modifications even as vital, and have a laugh each milestone along the manner.

Nutrition and Hydration for Endurance Running

Proper nutrients and hydration are critical for patience runners, particularly for older adults who may additionally have one in all a type nutritional desires. In this subchapter, we are able to discover the importance of vitamins and hydration for staying strength taking walks and provide sensible recommendations for older runners to optimize their general overall performance and acquainted health.

As we age, our our bodies go through various changes that may have an impact on our nutritional requirements. Older adults want to cognizance on ingesting a balanced eating regimen that consists of a whole lot of nutrient-dense meals. This manner incorporating carbohydrates, proteins, healthful fats, nutrients, and minerals into their food.

Carbohydrates are specially vital for staying electricity runners as they offer the number one supply of gasoline for muscle corporations in the course of prolonged-distance runs. It is commonly endorsed to eat complex carbohydrates which incorporates whole grains, end result, and vegetables for sustained electricity. Additionally, protein is essential for muscle restore and recovery, so older runners must cause to encompass lean property of protein like fowl, fish, beans, and nuts in their weight-reduction plan.

Hydration is a few different key detail of persistence on foot, as dehydration can negatively impact overall performance and boom the risk of injury. Older adults need to drink water often within the route of the day and boom their fluid intake in advance than, in a few unspecified time within the destiny of, and after their runs. Electrolyte-wealthy liquids also can assist top off misplaced minerals and preserve proper hydration degrees.

To ensure most useful vitamins and hydration, older runners ought to keep in mind the timing of their meals and snacks. It is usually recommended to devour a balanced meal containing carbohydrates, protein, and healthy fat a few hours in advance than a long time. During the run, ingesting small portions of with out problem digestible carbohydrates, which includes power gels or sports activities drinks, can assist preserve energy levels. After the run, a aggregate of carbohydrates and protein must be fed on to useful useful resource in muscle restoration.

Chapter 2: Running Gear and Equipment

Choosing the Right Running Shoes for Support and Comfort

When it involves taking walks, one of the most crucial factors to keep in thoughts is deciding on the right pair of walking footwear. As we age, our our bodies require greater resource and luxury to save you damage and make sure an fun strolling revel in. In this subchapter, we are capable of find out the important thing concerns for choosing strolling shoes that cater to the desires of older adults.

When deciding on walking shoes, it's far critical to prioritize support and cushioning. Look for footwear that provide good enough arch assist and cushioning in the heel and forefoot. This will assist take in the impact of each step, lowering the hazard of joint and muscle pressure. Additionally, older adults and people with particular foot situations, which include plantar fasciitis or bunions, have to choose footwear that provide extra help and accommodate the ones situations.

Comfort is every other essential element to don't forget. Make positive to strive on terrific producers and models to discover the suitable wholesome for your feet. Look for footwear with a roomy toe subject to keep away from cramped feet and functionality blisters. It is also advocated to choose out footwear with breathable substances to prevent excessive sweating and pain sooner or later of longer runs.

Furthermore, undergo in thoughts the sort of terrain you may be walking on. If you must run on trails or choppy surfaces, pick out direction taking walks shoes that provide stronger balance and traction. These footwear have a extra rugged outsole and brought protection to navigate thru rocks, roots, and other limitations.

Finally, it's miles essential to replace your walking footwear regularly. As a popular rule, walking shoes want to get replaced each 3 hundred-500 miles or every six months, depending on your frequency of use. Over time, the cushioning and useful resource in shoes placed on out, that may bring about ache and multiplied hazard of harm.

In give up, choosing the proper on foot footwear is of maximum significance for older adults. Prioritizing manual, cushioning, consolation, and suitability for the terrain will make certain an a laugh and stable on foot enjoy. Remember to replace your footwear regularly to preserve maximum excessive satisfactory standard overall performance and save you damage. Happy running!

Apparel and Accessories for Optimal Performance

When it involves strolling, having the proper garb and accessories have to make a international of distinction, especially for older adults. Whether you are a pro marathoner or actually beginning out, making an investment in the right gadget can beautify your regular overall performance, save you accidents, and make your runs more interesting. In this subchapter, we are capable of discover the important strolling garb and accessories which is probably specifically designed for people over forty.

One of the maximum important portions of tools for older runners is a first rate pair of walking shoes. As we age, our toes and joints end up more liable to harm, so it's critical to choose more than one footwear that offer sufficient cushioning and assist. Look for footwear with extra padding, arch assist, and a massive toe box to residence any foot troubles or swelling that can upward thrust up.

In addition to footwear, compression socks or sleeves may be a sport-changer for older runners. These tight-becoming garments enhance blood flow into, reduce muscle soreness, and offer greater aid to the calves. They also can help save you not unusual troubles like shin splints and Achilles tendonitis.

Another have to-have accessory for older runners is a well-becoming sports sports bra for women. As we age, our breast tissue can emerge as lots less employer, making it critical to find out a bra that gives proper useful resource and stops pain at some stage in runs. Look for bras with adjustable straps and a massive band below the bust for optimum consolation and balance.

When it includes clothing, moisture-wicking and breathable fabric are key. These materials assist to alter frame temperature and maintain you dry, preventing chafing and pain. Opt for mild-weight, short-drying tops and bottoms that permit for a complete style of motion. Additionally, bear in thoughts investing in reflective equipment or apparel with reflective accents to beautify visibility for the duration of early morning or midnight runs.

Finally, maintain in mind the significance of accessories like hats, solar sunglasses, and sunscreen. Protecting yourself from the sun's risky rays is vital, specifically for humans over forty, who can also have greater sensitive pores and pores and skin. Choose a massive-brimmed hat, UV-blocking off sunglasses, and a sweat-resistant sunscreen to defend yourself from the factors.

By equipping your self with the right apparel and add-ons, you'll be setting yourself up for success as an older runner. Not simplest will you revel in extra cushty and confident in the end of your runs, but you may also be taking crucial steps toward damage prevention and highest quality normal universal performance. So do not underestimate the energy of right tool – it is able to clearly make a difference to your on foot adventure.

Safety Gear and Technology for Older Runners

As we age, it becomes an increasing number of essential to prioritize safety while undertaking physical sports along with on foot. Fortunately, there are numerous protection system and era alternatives to be had that would help older runners live steady and prevent accidents. In this subchapter, we're capable of find out a number of the ones options and speak their benefits for older adults.

One of the most crucial protection gears for older runners is a good pair of taking walks shoes. As we age, our ft go through modifications, together with a lower in cushioning and arch useful resource. Therefore, it's far essential to put money into footwear that offer adequate surprise absorption and stability. Look for footwear mainly designed for older runners, which frequently function more cushioning and help.

Another safety equipment that can notably advantage older runners is a reflective vest or apparel. As visibility turns into more tough with age, carrying reflective equipment can help increase visibility to motorists and specific runners, mainly all through low-slight conditions. This is particularly essential for folks who experience strolling early inside the morning or past due within the middle of the night.

Technology additionally plays a massive function in improving safety for older runners. One such era is smartwatches or fitness trackers. These gadgets can track your coronary heart rate, distance, tempo, or perhaps ship indicators in case of any irregularities. They moreover embody GPS skills, which may be beneficial whilst on foot in unfamiliar areas or trails.

In addition to smartwatches, there also are safety apps available which can provide a in addition layer of safety for older runners. These apps will let you percentage your place with trusted contacts, ship distress signs, or even provide emergency offerings with vital scientific facts. Some apps additionally come with capabilities like a virtual running pal or guided bodily sports, which may be motivating and exciting.

Chapter 3: Running Injury Prevention

Common Running Injuries and How to Avoid Them

Running is a outstanding shape of exercising that would assist older adults, veterans, parents, grandparents, experts, and health lovers hold their physical and highbrow well-being. However, it is vital to be aware about commonplace walking accidents that could rise up, specially for humans over forty. By taking preventative measures, you could keep to revel in the benefits of running with out the hazard of damage.

One not unusual walking harm is shin splints, which cause pain alongside the the the front of the decrease leg. To keep away from this, it is critical to regularly growth your mileage and depth, placed on proper strolling shoes with particular cushioning and help, and make certain you have got right taking walks shape. It is likewise advocated to boost your lower leg muscles via wearing sports like calf increases and toe taps.

Another commonplace damage is runner's knee, which motives pain throughout the kneecap. To prevent this, it's miles vital to boost the muscle groups across the knee, inclusive of the quadriceps and hamstrings, thru sports like squats and lunges. It is also important to take note of your body and keep away from overtraining, as this may result in imbalances and elevated stress on the knee.

Plantar fasciitis is a situation characterised via way of pain inside the heel or arch of the foot. To avoid this, it's miles important to put on footwear with suitable arch assist and cushioning, stretch the calf and foot muscle companies in advance than and after taking walks, and often growth your mileage and intensity.

Achilles tendonitis is each other harm that would arise from strolling. To prevent this, it's miles essential to reinforce the calf muscle businesses via physical games like heel raises and to keep away from excessive hill taking walks or abrupt will increase in mileage or depth.

To keep away from those and one-of-a-kind strolling accidents, it's miles encouraged to concentrate to your frame and take relaxation days whilst desired. Incorporating move-schooling activities, at the side of swimming or cycling, can also help to prevent overuse accidents and decorate popular health. It is crucial to warmness up earlier than every run and cool down in a while, along side stretching sports activities for the primary muscle agencies concerned in jogging.

By following those preventative measures and being conscious of your frame's desires, you can maintain to experience the severa blessings of on foot without the risk of common accidents. Remember, running should be a lifelong pursuit, and looking after your body is crucial for lengthy-time period achievement and leisure in the game.

Warm-up and Cool-down Techniques for Injury Prevention

As we age, it will become increasingly more crucial to attend to our our our bodies and prevent accidents whilst undertaking physical sports sports like taking walks. One manner to do this is thru incorporating proper warm-up and funky-down techniques into our exercising workouts. These strategies now not handiest assist save you accidents but also beautify general universal overall performance and popular nicely-being. In this subchapter, we can talk a few effective warmness-up and funky-down techniques specifically tailor-made for humans over forty.

To start, permit's dive into the importance of warming up in advance than a run. A proper heat-up prepares your frame for the bodily goals of taking walks, will growth blood float to your muscle organizations, and complements flexibility. Begin with a few mild aerobic bodily sports which encompass brisk on foot or cycling for approximately 5-10 minutes. This helps growth your coronary heart charge regularly and warms up your muscle mass. Afterward, include dynamic stretches that target major muscle groups, along with leg swings, arm circles, and lunges. These actions assist to enhance variety of movement and spark off the muscle groups you'll be using within the route of your run.

Once you've finished your run, it's vital to relax well to aid in the recuperation system and reduce muscle discomfort. Slow down your pace little by little and have interaction in a couple of minutes of low-intensity jogging or strolling. This facilitates step by step lower your coronary heart rate and save you blood pooling on your legs. Following this, carry out static stretches, preserving each stretch for approximately 20-30 seconds. Focus on stretching your calves, quadriceps, hamstrings, and hip flexors. This will assist decorate flexibility and prevent muscle imbalances.

While warmth-up and funky-down techniques are important, it's far similarly important to pay interest to your body and modify them consequently. As we age, our our our bodies may additionally require greater time to warmth up or sit back out, so take the essential time to perform that. Additionally, if you have any pre-gift situations or accidents, are looking for recommendation from a healthcare professional or an authorized trainer for customized warmth-up and funky-down sporting events.

Incorporating those warm-up and cool-down strategies into your strolling habitual could make a good sized difference in damage prevention, performance enhancement, and regular nicely-being. By taking a few more minutes in advance than and after your run, you are making an funding to your extended-term health and ensuring that you may keep walking strong properly into your 40s and beyond.

Rehabilitation and Recovery Strategies for Older Runners

Chapter 4: The Role of Running in Weight Management

Maintaining a healthy weight will become increasingly more critical as we age. Excess weight can purpose severa fitness troubles, together with coronary heart sickness, diabetes, and joint issues. While there are numerous strategies to govern weight, strolling has established to be an effective and available approach for older adults.

Running is a notably green manner to burn calories and growth metabolism. As we age, our metabolism definitely slows down, making weight control greater hard. Regular walking can assist counteract this effect thru revving up your metabolism and increasing calorie expenditure, even at the equal time as at relaxation. By mission ordinary running periods, older adults can create a calorie deficit, essential to weight loss and improved frame composition.

Moreover, going for walks offers particular advantages for weight manipulate in comparison to exceptional varieties of workout. Running is a weight-bearing exercising, this means that it locations pressure for your bones and muscle organizations, which allows to keep and decorate bone density, lowering the danger of osteoporosis. Additionally, walking is a excessive-effect hobby that requires large power expenditure, making it alternatively powerful for burning strength and dropping unwanted pounds.

Running furthermore promotes the maintenance of lean muscle groups, that is essential for weight manipulate. As we age, we in fact lose muscles, that would slow down metabolism and reason weight gain. By incorporating walking into your ordinary, you may help maintain and construct muscle, leading to a better resting metabolic price and superior weight control.

Furthermore, walking has a best effect on highbrow and emotional well-being, that couldn't at once contribute to weight manage. Regular runners regularly enjoy a discount in stress tiers, progressed mood, and accelerated self-self guarantee. These highbrow benefits can help save you emotional ingesting and promote healthier food choices, ultimately assisting in weight manipulate.

To make the most of walking for weight control, it's far vital to mix it with a balanced food regimen. Running by myself cannot atone for a bad diet regime. Ensure you fuel your body with nutrient-dense materials that support your strolling ordinary and weight manage goals.

In stop, taking walks performs a important function in weight manage for older adults. It gives a mess of benefits, which include stepped forward calorie expenditure, improved body composition, renovation of lean muscle tissues, and greater suitable intellectual and emotional properly-being. By incorporating walking into your habitual and adopting a balanced healthy eating plan, you may attain and hold a healthy weight, reduce the danger of persistent sicknesses, and improve simple extremely good of lifestyles.

Nutrition and Exercise Strategies for Sustainable Weight Loss

When it comes to weight loss, the secret is to recognition on sustainable techniques that sell extended-term success. In this subchapter, we can discover nutrients and exercise strategies especially tailor-made for human beings over 40 who are seeking to lose weight and maintain a healthy frame composition.

Nutrition plays a critical feature in weight manipulate, specially as we age. As older adults, veterans, parents, grandparents, and professionals, it's miles important to prioritize nutrient-dense food that provide essential nutrients, minerals, and antioxidants. Incorporating a balanced food plan rich in lean proteins, complete grains, culmination, veggies, and wholesome fat can assist assist weight reduction efforts.

Additionally, detail manipulate is crucial for sustainable weight reduction. Paying interest to thing sizes and going for walks in the direction of conscious consuming can prevent overconsumption and promote a healthful metabolism. It is also encouraged to limit processed elements, sugary snacks, and drinks excessive in introduced sugars, as they could contribute to weight benefit and prevent improvement.

In conjunction with proper nutrients, normal workout is important for sustainable weight loss. Running is an high-quality form of workout for humans over forty, as it no longer most effective burns energy however furthermore promotes cardiovascular health, joint power, and intellectual nicely-being.

To begin a strolling software application, it's miles critical to visit a healthcare professional, specially when you have any pre-present conditions. Gradually growth your mileage and intensity to prevent accidents and allow your body to conform. Incorporating a mixture of staying electricity runs, pace exercises, and power training sporting occasions can maximize weight reduction and decorate body composition.

In terms of fueling your runs, motive to consume a balanced meal or snack containing carbohydrates and protein approximately 1-2 hours earlier than your workout. This will provide your frame with the important electricity to hold your run and aid in muscle recovery.

After your run, attention on replenishing your body with nutrient-dense elements and hydrating effectively. This will assist muscle healing, reduce contamination, and optimize your weight loss efforts.

Remember, sustainable weight reduction is a adventure that calls for staying power, consistency, and a holistic approach. By combining a healthful, balanced diet plan with ordinary strolling and exercising, people over 40 can collect their weight reduction goals on the same time as improving regular health, strength levels, and nicely-being.

Building Lean Muscle and Boosting Metabolism Through Running

Running is an first rate form of workout for human beings over 40 who're seeking to construct lean muscle and decorate their metabolism. Not most effective does walking offer a cardiovascular exercising, but it additionally engages a couple of muscle agencies, helping to strengthen and tone the body.

One of the important issue advantages of going for walks for older adults is its capability to increase lean muscle tissues. As we age, we definitely lose muscle tissues, which can result in a decrease in metabolism and an growth in body fats. However, by means of using manner of incorporating strolling into our health ordinary, we can counteract this muscle loss and keep a wholesome body composition.

Running is a weight-bearing exercising, that means that it locations strain at the bones, which enables to assemble and preserve bone density. This is specially important for older adults who are at a higher chance of developing osteoporosis. By task regular on foot, individuals can help their bones and reduce the hazard of fractures and other bone-associated accidents.

In addition to building lean muscle and improving bone density, on foot additionally has a remarkable impact on metabolism. The extra lean muscle businesses we've got were given, the greater energy our our our our bodies burn at rest. This is due to the reality muscle calls for more energy to keep than fats. By incorporating walking into our fitness regular, we can boom our popular muscle groups, which in flip boosts our metabolism and allows us burn extra energy all through the day.

To maximize the blessings of strolling for building lean muscle and boosting metabolism, it is crucial to comprise power training carrying sports into our habitual. Strength schooling sports activities sports, such as squats, lunges, and push-ups, assist to similarly give a boost to and tone the muscle groups. By combining walking with electricity training, humans can attain maximum suitable consequences in phrases of muscle growth and metabolism boosting.

In prevent, strolling is an extraordinary form of workout for older adults searching for to bring together lean muscle and boom their metabolism. By incorporating strolling into our fitness regular and mixing it with electricity education sports, we will benefit a strong and toned body at the same time as moreover improving our common health and well-being. Whether you are a beginner or an skilled runner, it's far in no manner too late to begin reaping the benefits of walking for muscle increase and metabolism boosting.

Chapter 5: Running Programs and Workouts

Starting a Running Program Safely and Effectively

Are you over 40 and on the lookout for to begin a jogging utility? Congratulations! Running is a notable way to enhance your bodily and highbrow properly-being, and it's far in no way too past due to start. However, it's far vital to method strolling with warning, especially as we age. In this subchapter, we are succesful to talk approximately a manner to begin a walking utility appropriately and successfully, deliberating the correct desires of older adults.

Before you lace up your walking footwear, it is crucial to talk over together together with your healthcare provider, especially when you have any pre-modern clinical situations. They can provide precious guidance and ensure that on foot is stable for you.

Once you have obtained the inexperienced mild, it's time to start slowly and regularly boom your walking amount. This is specially crucial for older adults, as our our bodies take longer to get better. Begin with a combination of taking walks and taking walks, regularly increasing the time spent taking walks and decreasing the time spent on foot. This will assist your body adapt to the demands of strolling and decrease the chance of damage.

Investing in right walking equipment and device is likewise important. Older runners may additionally moreover benefit from footwear with extra cushioning to lower the impact on joints. Additionally, recall using compression socks or sleeves to assist movement and decrease muscle soreness.

Injuries can appear to all people, but they'll be in particular negative for human beings over 40. To save you accidents, contain power training carrying occasions into your ordinary. Strengthening the muscle mass that help your joints can enhance balance and reduce the threat of strains or sprains.

As you improvement for your taking walks program, hold a watch constant constant to your frame composition and weight loss dreams. Running may be an remarkable tool for dropping pounds and enhancing body composition, but it's essential to gasoline your frame properly. Make high-quality to consume a balanced weight loss plan that consists of masses of end result, greens, lean proteins, and entire grains.

Running isn't pretty a lot physical health; it furthermore has numerous intellectual and emotional benefits. Many human beings over 40 discover that running helps reduce strain, enhance temper, and improve regular properly-being. Consider incorporating mindfulness strategies or running with a pal to beautify the intellectual blessings of your running software program.

Lastly, do not be afraid to discover new jogging evaluations. Trail walking and outdoor adventures can provide a clean exchange of environment and challenge your body in special strategies. Just make sure which you have the best device and take critical precautions on the equal time as venturing off-road.

Remember, starting a going for walks software is a journey, now not a holiday spot. Listen in your body, be patient with your self, and characteristic amusing small victories along the manner. With proper care and interest, going for walks can be a lifelong ardour that brings you delight, health, and strength.

Interval Training and Progression for Beginners

Interval education is a pretty effective approach of improving cardiovascular health and staying energy, making it a tremendous method for novices looking for to begin a strolling software program. This subchapter will guide older adults, veterans, mother and father, grandparents, specialists, and health enthusiasts through the fundamentals of c programming language schooling and the way to improvement efficaciously and efficiently.

Interval schooling includes alternating periods of immoderate-intensity exercising with durations of lower-intensity recuperation or relaxation. For novices, it's far critical to begin with viable intervals and often increase the intensity and period through the years. This permits the body to conform and prevent damage.

To begin, pick out out a steady and flat going for walks floor, in conjunction with a song or a treadmill. Warm up with a brisk stroll or moderate jog for five-10 minutes to put together the muscle mass and joints for exercise. Then, begin with a easy c language exercise: exchange among 1 minute of strolling or on foot at a mild tempo and 1 minute of taking walks or slow taking walks for healing. Repeat this cycle for a whole of 10-15 minutes.

As you turn out to be more comfortable with the initial exercising, regularly boom the period of the jogging durations and decrease the recuperation time. For instance, you may improvement to taking walks for 2 mins and convalescing for 30 seconds. Aim to finish three-four devices of those longer periods.

It is crucial to pay interest to your frame and no longer push too hard too speedy. If you enjoy any ache or pain, take a harm and discuss with a healthcare expert or going for walks train. Remember, the aim is to progress often and punctiliously.

To similarly enhance your c programming language training, consider incorporating hills or inclines into your exercising workouts. This will upload a similarly venture and interact one-of-a-type muscle businesses. Additionally, strive numerous the depth of your high-intensity intervals through growing your tempo or incorporating quick bursts of sprinting.

As you still development with c programming language training, it's far vital to incorporate rest days into your agenda to permit your body to get better and adapt. This will help save you overuse accidents and beautify regular preferred overall performance.

In cease, c language education is an tremendous tool for novices over forty who are looking for to enhance their cardiovascular health and staying power. By starting with potential periods and steadily growing the depth and duration, you could competently improvement and gather the blessings of this education approach. Remember to continuously deal with your frame, incorporate rest days, and talk with a professional if desired. Get geared up to take your walking to the subsequent diploma and experience the numerous benefits it brings on your common health and well-being.

Incorporating Strength and Cross-Training for Overall Fitness

As you age, it turns into even extra crucial to prioritize common health and nicely-being. Running on my own won't be sufficient to preserve a wholesome and lively way of life.

That's in which incorporating power and go-education into your ordinary ought to make a big distinction. In this subchapter, we are able to find out the blessings of incorporating electricity and pass-training physical activities for human beings over forty.

Strength training is critical for older adults because it allows maintain and construct muscle tissue, which actually declines with age. By incorporating strength sporting sports into your regular, you can increase your electricity, enhance your stability, and decrease the risk of falls. These sports activities activities can be as smooth as bodyweight squats, lunges, push-ups, or the use of resistance bands or dumbbells. By little by little growing the depth and resistance, you may mission your muscle agencies and promote boom and improvement.

Cross-training, however, entails venture one-of-a-type forms of sports activities or bodily video games that complement your going for walks routine. It facilitates to prevent overuse injuries, as it reduces the repetitive stress that walking locations to your joints and muscle tissue. Cross-schooling sports activities sports can embody swimming, biking, yoga, Pilates, or perhaps dancing. These sports no longer most effective offer a smash from taking walks but moreover improve flexibility, core energy, and cardiovascular fitness.

By incorporating strength and bypass-schooling into your recurring, you may experience numerous advantages. First and maximum important, it is able to assist prevent injuries with the aid of using strengthening your muscle corporations and improving your body's everyday sturdiness. It furthermore enhances your on foot normal performance with the aid of manner of improving your pace, staying energy, and form. Additionally, cross-schooling can provide intellectual and emotional well-being, because it affords range and entertainment to your health ordinary.

To contain power and move-training successfully, it is essential to have a properly-rounded exercise plan. This consists of allocating unique days for energy schooling and incorporating flow into-schooling sports activities to your non-taking walks days. It is likewise important to pay attention for your body, relaxation whilst desired, and are looking for steering from a fitness professional or teacher if important.

In stop, incorporating power and pass-schooling physical sports into your normal as an older person might also want to have severa advantages. By that specialize in ordinary health, you can preserve and enhance your bodily strength, save you injuries, and decorate your strolling average performance. Remember, it's miles in no manner too beyond because of start incorporating those sports activities into your ordinary, and the rewards will be well without a doubt well worth the effort.

Chapter 6: Running and Maintaining Joint Health

Understanding Joint Health and Aging

As we age, it will become increasingly more essential to attend to our joints, especially for the ones oldsters which are enthusiastic about strolling. Joint fitness plays a crucial role in our capability to preserve on foot properly into our 40s and beyond. In this subchapter, we are able to delve into the intricacies of joint fitness and growing antique, exploring the elements that have an impact on our joints and the way we're able to maintain their fitness as we turn out to be older.

One of the critical element components to recognize is the natural growing older approach and its impact on our joints. As we age, the cartilage that cushions our joints begins to wear down, important to situations which embody osteoarthritis. This can purpose pain, stiffness, and decreased mobility, making it important to take proactive measures to assist joint fitness.

Regular workout, together with running, can in fact be useful for our joints. It enables to strengthen the muscle mass that surround and resource the joints, lowering the stress positioned on them. However, it's far critical to strike a stability and avoid overtraining, as immoderate stress on the joints can cause harm and long-term harm.

In addition to exercise, proper nutrients is vital for retaining joint fitness. Consuming a weight loss program rich in anti-inflammatory meals, which incorporates cease stop result, veggies, whole grains, and fatty fish, can assist reduce irritation inside the joints. It's additionally important to stay hydrated, as water permits lubricate the joints and preserve them functioning optimally.

Furthermore, incorporating rest and restoration into our walking ordinary is important for joint fitness. Giving our bodies time to get better amongst runs permits the joints to restore and rebuild, decreasing the risk of overuse injuries. Additionally, the usage of strategies together with stretching, foam rolling, and regular massages can help alleviate muscle anxiety and enhance joint mobility.

Lastly, it is critical to concentrate to our our our bodies and are looking for professional assist if we enjoy persistent joint pain or discomfort. Consulting a healthcare expert, which includes a physiotherapist or orthopedic professional, can help diagnose any underlying troubles and offer suitable remedy alternatives.

By information the impact of growing older on our joints and imposing techniques to help their health, we can keep to revel in the benefits of jogging well into our 40s and beyond. Taking care of our joints no longer only allows us to preserve an active way of life however additionally contributes to our not unusual bodily and intellectual well-being.

Exercises and Stretches for Joint Mobility and Flexibility

As we age, keeping joint mobility and flexibility becomes increasingly more essential. Whether you are an older character, a veteran, a determine, a grandparent, a expert, or in reality a health fanatic, incorporating wearing sports and stretches into your routine can drastically advantage your everyday properly-being. In this subchapter, we will find out severa sporting events and stretches specially designed for human beings over 40, specializing of their joint health, mobility, and versatility.

Regular exercise and stretching can help save you joint stiffness, lessen the chance of accidents, and beautify your commonplace preferred performance, whether you're a pro runner or certainly starting out. The physical activities and stretches outlined on this subchapter are mainly tailored to cope with the desires of runners over 40, thinking about the perfect challenges they'll face.

You will studies some of wearing activities that focus on unique joints, along side the hips, knees, ankles, and shoulders. These sports activities will assist decorate your joint mobility, contemplating a more form of motion and lowering the threat of joint ache or stiffness. Additionally, you can discover diverse stretches that focus on developing flexibility within the muscles surrounding those joints.

Incorporating the ones sports activities and stretches into your ordinary ordinary ought to have severa blessings. They can beautify your taking walks overall overall performance, permitting you to increase your pace and patience. They also can reduce the danger of accidents, consisting of sprains or lines, which may be extra not unusual as we age. Furthermore, the ones bodily sports and stretches can help alleviate joint ache and ache, permitting you to keep taking element inside the physical sports you want.

Whether you're embarking on a marathon education software, seeking to shed pounds, or honestly trying to maintain your joint health, this subchapter will provide you with valuable insights and practical sporting activities to integrate into your every day routine. By prioritizing joint mobility and versatility, you may decorate your strolling revel in, improve your common properly-being, and hold to steer an active and notable lifestyles.

Remember, it is never too late to begin prioritizing your joint health. With the proper sports activities and stretches, you can preserve your mobility and flexibility, permitting you to enjoy the benefits of strolling nicely into your golden years. So, permit's get started out and discover the sporting activities and stretches that will help you keep sturdy and bendy joints for future years!

Joint-Friendly Running Surfaces and Techniques

As we age, it turns into more and more essential to take care of our joints, mainly at the same time as sporting out physical sports activities like strolling. Joint-pleasant taking walks surfaces and strategies can assist lessen the hazard of damage and make sure that we will hold to experience the benefits of strolling nicely into our golden years. In this subchapter, we are capable of discover a number of the pleasant practices for older adults, veterans, mother and father, grandparents, professionals, and fitness enthusiasts who are inquisitive about walking over forty.

Chapter 7: Mental and Emotional Well-Being in Individuals

The Psychological Benefits of Running for Older Adults

Running is a top notch physical activity that offers severa advantages for people of each age. For older adults, in particular, walking ought to have large intellectual advantages that make contributions to common properly-being and first-rate of lifestyles. In this subchapter, we delve into the mental advantages of going for walks for older adults, highlighting how it can undoubtedly impact intellectual and emotional health.

One of the vital component mental advantages of on foot for older adults is stress cut price. Running affords a herbal outlet for freeing pressure and tension, allowing the mind to unwind and loosen up. Engaging in everyday going for walks intervals can help older adults address the everyday traumatic conditions and pressures of lifestyles, selling a feel of calmness and calmness.

Running moreover performs a important feature in boosting mood and combating signs and signs and signs of despair and anxiety. The release of endorphins sooner or later of workout can create a euphoric feeling commonly known as the "runner's excessive." This herbal mood enhancer can deliver spirits, growth self-self guarantee, and enhance common intellectual nicely-being.

Moreover, taking walks can enhance cognitive characteristic and thoughts health in older adults. Studies have verified that normal aerobic workout, along with going for walks, can enhance reminiscence, hobby, and trouble-solving capabilities. Running promotes the growth of new brain cells and improves blood drift to the mind, resulting in greater high quality cognitive typical usual performance and decreased risk of cognitive decline.

Participating in strolling can also foster a enjoy of accomplishment and decorate vanity in older adults. Achieving personal walking dreams, which embody finishing a race or growing distance, can provide a experience of cause and fulfillment. This may be specially empowering for older adults who can be managing challenges associated with growing vintage.

Lastly, on foot offers an opportunity for social connection and interplay. Joining strolling organizations or participating in neighborhood races lets in older adults to have interaction with like-minded people, fostering a feel of community and camaraderie. This social issue of strolling can combat emotions of loneliness and isolation, selling everyday mental well-being.

In stop, walking offers a multitude of highbrow advantages for older adults. From stress discount and mood enhancement to advanced cognitive function and social connection, taking walks is a valuable device for selling highbrow and emotional nicely-being. By incorporating on foot into their lives, older adults can revel in a renewed experience of strength and revel in the endless rewards that strolling has to offer.

Stress Reduction and Mental Clarity Through Running

In ultra-modern speedy-paced and disturbing global, pressure is a common trouble that affects human beings of each age. However, as we age, it turns into even more crucial to find out effective strategies to control pressure and maintain highbrow clarity. Fortunately, walking can be a powerful tool for pressure discount and selling intellectual nicely-being, in particular for human beings over 40.

Running is a herbal pressure reliever, because it lets in release endorphins, furthermore known as the "revel in-amazing" hormones. These hormones interact with receptors in the thoughts, reducing feelings of ache and stress and selling a revel in of euphoria. Engaging in normal walking intervals can considerably reduce tension, melancholy, and fashionable strain degrees.

Additionally, jogging presents a much-wanted break out from the every day pressures and duties of life. It lets in older adults, veterans, mother and father, grandparents, experts, and health enthusiasts to take time for themselves, disconnect from shows and duties, and consciousness on their very very own bodily and mental well-being. This time of solitude and introspection can lead to greater suitable highbrow readability and the capability to count on more definitely and creatively.

Moreover, going for walks offers an opportunity to exercise mindfulness, a way that includes focusing one's interest on the winning 2nd. By concentrating at the rhythm of your breath, the sensation of your toes hitting the ground, and the sounds of nature, you could cultivate a feel of intellectual clarity and internal calm. This mindfulness exercising in the direction of strolling can assist older individuals find peace, lessen bad mind, and decorate everyday intellectual well-being.

Furthermore, going for walks may be an notable outlet for releasing pent-up feelings and frustrations. As you push yourself bodily, you may additionally release highbrow tension and strain. The repetitive movement of jogging may be meditative, permitting you to method feelings and advantage a easy mind-set on existence's traumatic situations. It gives a enjoy of success and boosts self-self belief, fundamental to advanced mental resilience.

In give up, strolling is a effective tool for stress cut price and intellectual clarity, especially for humans over 40. By venture regular walking durations, older adults can revel in the benefits of progressed endorphins, extra effective highbrow readability, advanced mindfulness, and emotional release. Whether you are a novice or an skilled runner, incorporating going for walks into your normal can have a profound impact to your standard properly-being, assisting you navigate the traumatic situations of existence with extra ease and readability.

Incorporating Mindfulness and Meditation into Your Running Practice

As we age, it becomes an increasing number of crucial to no longer simplest interest on our physical properly-being however moreover on our intellectual and emotional health. The exercising of mindfulness and meditation has gained full-size popularity in current years, and for true motive. It has been shown to reduce stress, decorate awareness, and sell ordinary well-being. When mixed with the bodily benefits of jogging, mindfulness and meditation may be a effective tool for older adults trying to decorate their walking workout.

Mindfulness is the exercising of being attentive to the triumphing second, with out judgment. It includes absolutely immersing yourself within the revel in of walking, being aware about your breath, the sensation of your toes hitting the floor, and the factors of hobby and sounds spherical you. By bringing your interest to the prevailing 2d, you could permit move of the issues and distractions of everyday life, permitting yourself to simply revel in and admire your run.

Meditation, on the other hand, consists of setting aside devoted time to sit down down quietly and attention on your breath or a selected object of meditation. It may be a wonderful complement on your walking exercise, because it allows to calm the thoughts, enhance awareness, and reduce pressure. By incorporating meditation into your habitual, you may cultivate a experience of inner peace and highbrow readability, which can decorate your walking typical performance and cutting-edge nicely-being.

To encompass mindfulness and meditation into your taking walks workout, start thru putting aside a few minutes in advance than and after every run to exercise deep respiratory and aware reputation. Take a few deep breaths, specializing in the sensation of the breath coming into and leaving your frame. As you run, try to stay gift and clearly have interaction together with your environment. Notice the sensation of your toes hitting the floor, the rhythm of your breath, and the beauty of nature spherical you.

You also can take a look at with guided meditation apps or podcasts in particular designed for runners. These can offer you with guided mindfulness and meditation practices that you may be aware of whilst strolling. This can assist to keep you centered and present, even in the course of longer runs or difficult exercise workout routines.

Chapter 8: Cardiovascular Health and Disease Prevention in Those over Forty

The Cardiovascular Benefits of Running for Older Adults

Running is often seen as a recreation for the more youthful, but it holds first-rate blessings for older adults as nicely. In reality, strolling can be a powerful tool in promoting cardiovascular fitness and preventing ailments that usually have an effect on human beings over forty. In this subchapter, we are able to discover the diverse methods wherein strolling can make a contribution to a greater healthy coronary coronary heart and frequent properly-being in older adults.

One of the crucial aspect blessings of walking for older adults is its amazing effect on cardiovascular fitness. Regular going for walks permits to enhance the coronary heart muscle, enhancing its overall performance and functionality to pump blood for the duration of the frame. This prolonged cardiovascular fitness reduces the hazard of developing coronary heart illness, high blood stress, and stroke – commonplace troubles for people in this age institution.

Furthermore, walking lets in to keep wholesome cholesterol levels. As we age, our levels of cholesterol will be inclined to upward push, growing the hazard of plaque buildup within the arteries. By challenge regular on foot, older adults can lower their LDL (bad) levels of cholesterol and boom their HDL (actual) ldl ldl cholesterol, which aids in eliminating plaque from the arteries.

Running additionally performs a important characteristic in maintaining a healthy weight, each other essential thing in cardiovascular fitness. As we age, our metabolism has a bent to gradual down, making weight manipulate extra difficult. Running not remarkable burns strength throughout the interest but moreover boosts metabolism, essential to persevered calorie burn even after the run. By incorporating jogging into their regular, older adults can effectively manipulate their weight and decrease the hazard of weight problems-associated coronary coronary heart conditions.

Additionally, strolling has been shown to enhance blood go along with the waft and flow into. The repetitive motion of walking permits to bolster blood vessels and beautify their flexibility, selling better blood drift to the heart and special organs. This improved circulate reduces the risk of blood clots and keeps the cardiovascular tool functioning optimally.

Furthermore, taking walks has immoderate fine consequences on highbrow and emotional nicely-being, each of which can be carefully related to cardiovascular health. Regular taking walks releases endorphins, the body's herbal temper-boosting chemical materials, selling a enjoy of nicely-being and reducing pressure and anxiety. These intellectual benefits contribute to a more fit coronary coronary heart and a discounted hazard of heart sickness.

In quit, on foot offers severa cardiovascular benefits for older adults. By incorporating walking into their ordinary, humans over 40 can improve their coronary coronary heart, preserve wholesome levels of cholesterol, manipulate weight, decorate blood float, and enhance their intellectual and emotional well-being. Running is a effective device in promoting cardiovascular health and stopping ailments, permitting older adults to maintain their strength and experience an lively life-style for future years.

Reducing the Risk of Heart Disease and Other Chronic Conditions

Taking care of your coronary heart and not unusual health turns into increasingly crucial as we age. Heart ailment and one of a kind continual situations can significantly impact our incredible of lifestyles, making it vital to prioritize preventive measures. Running, mainly for individuals over 40, can be an effective tool for decreasing the hazard of coronary heart disorder and wonderful chronic situations. In this subchapter, we are able to discover how on foot can beautify cardiovascular fitness, raise energy tiers, and help hold vast well-being.

Regular strolling has been tested to bolster the coronary coronary heart muscle corporations, decorate blood motion, and reduce blood strain. By carrying out this cardio workout, older adults can lessen the chance of developing coronary heart sickness and associated situations, which includes immoderate ldl ldl cholesterol and excessive blood strain. Running additionally aids in weight control, some different essential element in stopping coronary heart sickness. By dropping extra pounds and retaining a healthful weight, human beings can notably reduce their risk of coronary heart-related issues.

Apart from cardiovascular fitness, walking can also enhance highbrow and emotional well-being. Many older adults revel in expanded pressure tiers because of various life conditions. Running gives an outlet for stress, releasing endorphins that increase mood and promote a experience of well-being. It also can help combat signs of anxiety and melancholy, promoting highbrow readability and emotional balance.

In addition to coronary coronary coronary heart health, walking can make a contribution to accelerated power and electricity. As we age, it's miles not unusual to enjoy a decline in strength ranges. However, regular walking can counteract this via way of boosting metabolism, enhancing oxygen drift, and developing ordinary stamina. By incorporating taking walks into your regular, you may revel in a terrific growth in power, making each day activities experience greater achievable.

Furthermore, strolling can useful useful resource in weight loss and frame composition changes. For people over 40, preserving a healthy weight becomes increasingly important. Running is a quite powerful calorie-burning hobby which can help shed extra weight and assemble lean muscular tissues. With a steady on foot software and a balanced weight-reduction plan, older adults can achieve their weight loss dreams and beautify their body composition.

In end, going for walks is a powerful tool for decreasing the risk of coronary heart sickness and other chronic conditions in human beings over forty. By incorporating this aerobic exercising into your recurring, you could improve your coronary heart, enhance cardiovascular fitness, boom energy stages, and preserve normal well-being. The blessings of on foot amplify beyond bodily fitness, absolutely impacting highbrow and emotional properly-being as nicely. Prioritizing your coronary coronary coronary heart fitness and fashionable wellbeing via walking will contribute to a extra match, happier, and further pleasurable life.

Monitoring Heart Rate and Exercise Intensity for Optimal Cardiovascular Health

One of the critical component factors in attaining very last cardiovascular health through strolling is tracking your heart fee and exercise depth. This subchapter will discover the significance of tracking the ones metrics and the way they can help you maximize your exercise exercises and enhance your simple health.

As we age, our cardiovascular device genuinely undergoes changes, making it even greater vital to be aware of our coronary heart charge in the end of exercising. Older adults, veterans, mother and father, grandparents, experts, and fitness fans can all advantage from data how to expose their coronary heart rate efficiently.

By tracking your coronary coronary heart rate, you can make certain which you are workout inner your goal coronary coronary heart charge vicinity, this is the type of heartbeats in step with minute this is most useful for cardiovascular fitness. This region varies primarily based mostly on factors together with age and fitness degree.

To display display screen your coronary coronary heart rate all through exercise, you may use wearable devices together with coronary coronary heart rate monitors or smartwatches. These devices provide actual-time comments in your coronary heart price, allowing you to adjust your depth subsequently. Alternatively, you may manually degree your coronary heart rate via checking your pulse at super periods for the duration of your workout.

Understanding exercise intensity is also vital for optimizing cardiovascular fitness. Different levels of depth elicit exceptional physiological responses in the frame. By exercising at the precise intensity, you can beautify your cardiovascular endurance, burn strength, and enhance normal fitness.

There are numerous strategies to decide workout depth, which include the speak take a look at, score of perceived exertion (RPE), and coronary heart price zones. The communicate take a look at includes assessing your capability to keep a verbal exchange on the identical time as exercise. If you can without issue talk, you will be workout at a lower depth, while struggling to talk shows a higher intensity.

RPE is a scale that allows you to rate how tough you recognize your attempt to be throughout exercising. This subjective diploma can assist guide your intensity ranges. Heart rate zones, as stated earlier, provide a greater aim degree of workout depth based totally mostly on your coronary coronary coronary heart rate.

By monitoring your coronary coronary heart fee and exercise depth, you can ensure that you are strolling out on the right level in your goals and wellknown cardiovascular fitness. Whether you're a beginner searching out to beautify your fitness or a seasoned runner aiming for a marathon, information and monitoring the ones metrics will assist you're making the most of your exercising routines and advantage most beneficial cardiovascular fitness.

In the subsequent section, we are able to delve deeper into precise heart price zones and the way to apply them effectively for numerous strolling applications and goals.

Chapter 9: Running For Increased Energy

Boosting Energy Levels and Fighting Fatigue through Running

One of the crucial factor advantages of walking, especially for individuals over forty, is its functionality to decorate energy levels and combat fatigue. As we age, it becomes greater hard to hold excessive electricity levels in a few unspecified time inside the destiny of the day, but incorporating walking into your ordinary may need to make a excellent difference.

Regular strolling has been confirmed to increase electricity levels by way of enhancing cardiovascular feature, improving blood movement, and selling the release of endorphins, which might be herbal temper-boosting hormones. When you've got interplay in a walking session, your coronary coronary heart rate increases, pumping extra oxygen and nutrients on your muscle businesses and organs, leaving you feeling energized and revitalized.

Moreover, on foot helps combat fatigue through enhancing sleep extraordinary. Studies have mounted that regular exercise, which encompass taking walks, can beautify sleep styles, reducing the chance of insomnia and selling deeper, extra restorative sleep. By getting higher high-quality sleep, you'll awaken feeling extra refreshed and prepared to take on the day.

Running moreover offers intellectual and emotional blessings that make contributions to accelerated strength ranges. It is famous that exercise, which encompass walking, can lessen pressure and anxiety degrees, decorate mood, and lift highbrow readability. By clearing your mind and liberating tension via taking walks, you may revel in more energized and focused inside the direction of the day.

In addition to those enormous blessings, there are particular strategies and techniques that older adults can rent to maximise the energy-boosting effects of strolling. It is critical to start step by step and pay interest on your body, permitting for proper rest and restoration to save you overexertion and burnout. Incorporating strength training sporting sports along walking can also help assemble muscle electricity and persistence, enhancing everyday strength stages.

Furthermore, taking note of nutrients and hydration is critical for preserving energy ranges in the course of and after walking periods. Consuming a balanced food plan rich in complicated carbohydrates, lean proteins, and healthy fat will offer the critical gas for your runs and beneficial useful resource in put up-workout recuperation. Staying properly hydrated via manner of consuming enough water at some stage in the day and throughout your runs is likewise important for power renovation.

By incorporating strolling into your way of life and imposing these strategies, you may revel in expanded strength ranges and combat fatigue successfully. Running is a versatile interest that may be tailored to fit your needs, whether or not or no longer you are a beginner or an skilled runner. So, put on your on foot footwear, hit the pavement, and enjoy the benefits of increased energy and energy that going for walks can deliver on your existence.

Nutrition and Hydration Strategies for Energy Optimization

As we age, our our our bodies undergo severa changes that might have an effect on our strength ranges and widespread performance, mainly in relation to physical sports like walking. However, with the proper vitamins and hydration strategies, older adults can optimize their strength tiers to hold gambling the benefits of walking nicely into their 40s and past.

Proper nutrients plays a critical characteristic in fueling your body for jogging. As an older man or woman, it's miles crucial to consciousness on ingesting a properly-balanced food plan that consists of pretty a few nutrient-dense components.

Incorporating lean proteins, complete grains, end result, vegetables, and wholesome fat into your meals can provide the critical electricity and vitamins to assist your strolling desires.

Hydration is further crucial, as dehydration can cause fatigue and reduced primary overall performance. Older adults can also have a faded thirst sensation, making it essential to drink fluids often, even in case you do no longer experience thirsty. Aim to devour at the least eight cups of water in step with day, and growth your intake inside the direction of walking classes to replace fluids out of place thru sweat.

To optimize energy ranges, go through in mind timing your meals and snacks strategically around your jogging schedule. Consuming a small, balanced meal or snack rich in carbohydrates and protein about to a few hours earlier than your run can provide a ordinary supply of electricity. Additionally, fueling at some stage in longer runs with effortlessly digestible carbohydrates, collectively with strength gels or sports activities activities liquids, can help maintain your energy degrees.

Supplements can also play a function in optimizing power levels for older runners. Consult with a healthcare professional to determine when you have any nutrient deficiencies that may benefit from supplementation. Common dietary nutritional dietary supplements for runners embody omega-3 fatty acids for joint health, vitamins D for bone strength, and B nutrients for strength metabolism.

Remember, nutrients and hydration techniques are pretty individualized, so it's far crucial to concentrate for your frame and make adjustments as wanted. Keep a mag to music how one of a kind substances and fluids have an impact on your energy tiers in a few unspecified time inside the future of jogging and alter your technique in the end.

By imposing those nutrition and hydration techniques, older adults can optimize their energy tiers, ensuring they have got the energy and stamina to keep taking walks and playing the numerous blessings it brings.

Incorporating Rest and Recovery for Sustainable Energy

One of the maximum vital factors of running, especially for people over forty, is making sure proper rest and recuperation. As we age, our bodies require greater time to get over bodily hobby, and neglecting this vital element can bring about fatigue, damage, and burnout. This subchapter will discover the importance of rest and recuperation for sustainable strength and provide sensible hints for incorporating it into your running habitual.

Rest and recovery play a essential characteristic in keeping strength degrees and stopping fatigue. When we engage in bodily interest, our muscle organizations go through pressure and micro-tears, which need time to repair and rebuild. Without right enough relaxation, those muscles can become overworked and vulnerable to harm. Additionally, relaxation permits our our our our bodies to fill up electricity stores, regulate hormones, and restore intellectual focus. Incorporating normal relaxation days into your training time table can assist save you burnout and make sure prolonged-term power sustainability.

There are severa techniques to incorporate relaxation and restoration into your on foot routine. Firstly, it is essential to be aware of your frame and recognize signs of fatigue or overtraining. If you experience excessively tired, sore, or examine a decline in overall performance, it can be time to take a rest day. Additionally, maintain in thoughts incorporating lively restoration sports which incorporates yoga, stretching, or low-impact physical games like swimming or biking on your rest days.

Chapter 10: Trail Running and Outdoor Adventures

Exploring the Benefits of Trail Running for Older Adults

As we age, retaining an energetic way of existence turns into increasingly more crucial for our bodily and mental well-being. While there are numerous forms of workout to select from, direction strolling stands proud as an excellent possibility for older adults. In this subchapter, we're capable of delve into the severa benefits that path strolling can offer human beings over the age of forty.

One of the important aspect benefits of route walking is its low-effect nature. Unlike pounding the pavement on roads, jogging on trails offers a softer floor that is gentler on getting old joints. This makes it a in reality ideal desire for older adults who may be involved approximately joint fitness or who have experienced previous accidents. Furthermore, the uneven terrain of trails engages a much wider style of muscle tissues, presenting a greater balanced and effective workout.

In addition to physical advantages, route walking furthermore gives a massive sort of intellectual and emotional blessings. Spending time in nature has been established to reduce strain degrees and enhance temper, which may be particularly beneficial for older adults managing the pressures of every day life. Trail walking permits you to break out the noise and chaos of the town and immerse your self in the calming splendor of herbal environment.

Moreover, direction walking offers a revel in of journey and exploration that could reignite the satisfaction of physical hobby. Discovering new trails and tough your self with severa terrains can assist to preserve your workout routines sparkling and engaging. This is particularly vital for older adults who might also additionally war with motivation or boredom of their health sporting activities.

For those searching out cardiovascular fitness and illness prevention, route walking is an excellent preference. The aggregate of aerobic exercising and the herbal elements of course on foot can assist to enhance coronary heart health, decrease blood strain, and decrease the risk of continual diseases together with coronary heart sickness and diabetes.

Lastly, route strolling offers an opportunity to connect to like-minded human beings and assemble a experience of network. Many strolling businesses and golf equipment cater specifically to older adults, presenting a supportive surroundings for individuals to percentage their ardour for taking walks and the outdoor.

In end, trail taking walks is an wonderful desire for older adults looking for a form of workout this is every bodily and mentally stimulating. With its low-impact nature, intellectual and emotional benefits, cardiovascular benefits, and possibilities for adventure and network, path strolling is a first-rate desire for people over the age of forty. Lace up your taking walks shoes, hit the paths, and include the general range of advantages that trail jogging has to provide.

Safety Tips and Techniques for Trail Running

Trail taking walks is a exciting and invigorating interest that would offer a clean trade of environment from the same old avenue or treadmill runs. However, strolling on choppy terrain and in natural environments comes with its very own set of demanding situations and capability risks. To ensure a stable and exciting route taking walks revel in, it's far essential to comply with the ones protection hints and techniques specially tailored for older adults.

1. Choose appropriate shoes: Invest in a couple of route walking footwear that provide amazing grip, balance, and safety from rocks and debris. Look for abilities like aggressive tread patterns and strengthened toe caps.

2. Dress for the conditions: Wear moisture-wicking and breathable clothing that suits the climate. Layering is certainly beneficial to adjust to converting temperatures. Don't forget approximately a hat and sunglasses for solar protection.

three. Plan your route and inform others: Before heading out, research the direction you recommend to run and allow someone apprehend your meant course and estimated pass once more time. Carry a map or use a GPS device for navigation.

4. Start sluggish and grade by grade growth intensity: Trail walking calls for greater strive and engages specific muscular tissues than road jogging. Begin with shorter distances and step by step growth your mileage and intensity to keep away from overexertion and functionality injuries.

five. Keep an eye fixed fixed on the terrain: Stay centered at the trail in advance to assume any obstacles or changes in the direction. Watch out for tree roots, rocks, unfastened gravel, and choppy surfaces.

6. Stay hydrated and fueled: Carry water or a hydration percent to top off fluids sooner or later of your run. Pack strength gels or snacks to preserve your power ranges on longer path runs.

7. Pack essentials: Carry a small first useful useful resource package deal deal, a whistle for emergencies, and a totally charged cell cellular telephone. Additionally, if strolling in a ways off regions, recall wearing a light-weight emergency blanket or extra layers for warmth.

8. Pay interest to herbal international and nature: Respect the surroundings and stay alert for any possibly dangerous herbal international. Make noise to avoid unexpected animals and be informed approximately nearby flora and fauna and their behavior.

nine. Listen in your frame: If you revel in pain or ache while taking walks, do no longer push via it. Take breaks, walk if critical, and are searching out clinical interest if symptoms and signs and signs persist.

10. Practice proper direction etiquette: Yield to hikers and slower runners, apprehend personal property, and depart no trace via manner of the use of carrying out any trash or waste.

By following the ones safety guidelines and techniques, older adults, veterans, dad and mom, grandparents, professionals, health fans, and individuals inside the aforementioned niches can revel in the pleasure and serenity of path strolling at the equal time as minimizing the risks related to this outdoor adventure. Remember, protection ought to constantly be a pinnacle precedence at the same time as hitting the trails.

Planning and Preparing for Outdoor Running Adventures

When it involves strolling, there can be some element particular approximately taking your exercising workout routines exterior. The easy air, scenic perspectives, and enjoy of journey should make every run experience like a brand new and exciting enjoy. For older adults, veterans, dad and mom, grandparents, professionals, and health lovers, outside on foot adventures can provide a large number of blessings, from physical fitness to highbrow properly-being. In this subchapter, we're able to discover the important additives of planning and making equipped for those outdoor taking walks adventures, making sure a stable and fun revel in for people over forty.

Firstly, it's miles crucial to pick out out the proper place on your outside strolling journey. Consider your fitness level, preferences, and goals at the same time as selecting a route or route. Some older runners may also moreover decide on flat terrains, whilst others may also are seeking out greater hard routes. Research the location in advance, looking for records on elevation modifications, terrain sorts, and any capability dangers to ensure your protection.

Next, acquire the important system and tool on your journey. Older runners can also gain from making an funding in supportive jogging footwear that provide stability and cushioning to lessen the risk of accidents. Additionally, don't forget wearing moisture-wicking clothing to live dry and cushty, further to a hat and sunscreen for sun protection. Don't forget about approximately to deliver a water bottle or hydration % to live hydrated throughout your run.

Prioritizing damage prevention and recovery is crucial, mainly for individuals over forty. Incorporate dynamic heat-up physical games in advance than every run to prepare your muscle corporations and joints for the hobby. After your run, perform static stretches to decorate flexibility and aid in recuperation. It's also essential to concentrate on your frame and take relaxation days whilst needed to keep away from overuse injuries.

If weight reduction or body composition changes are your motive, out of doors jogging adventures may be an powerful tool. Combine your runs with a balanced and nutritious food regimen to maximise your results. Consult with a registered dietitian or nutritionist to increase a personalized plan that suits your needs and dreams.

To make the most of your outdoor taking walks adventures, consider becoming a member of a walking application or locating a taking walks pal. These connections can offer obligation, motivation, and the opportunity to research from skilled runners. Additionally, taking element in prepared races or activities can add a further degree of delight and task to your strolling adventures.

Chapter 11: Discovering the Freedom of Movement

Running, a clean act of putting one foot in the front of the alternative, has the energy to unlock a worldwide of satisfaction and freedom. Beyond its bodily benefits, taking walks transcends right into a transformative experience that connects us with our bodies, minds, and the arena round us. In this bankruptcy, we delve into the pleasure of taking walks, exploring the reasons why it captivates our spirits, the myriad of benefits it offers, and the essential connection amongst on foot and our innate sense of freedom.

From the instant we take our first steps as runners, we embark on a journey of discovery. The open street beckons us with its ensures of adventure, new horizons, and a experience of boundless exploration. As our ft contact the floor, we emerge as one with nature, feeling the earth beneath us and the wind closer to our pores and pores and skin.

Running gives us with the opportunity to interrupt out the confines of our every day sports and step right proper right into a realm of countless opportunities. Whether it's a leisurely jog through a park or an invigorating sprint alongside a rugged course, running permits us to interrupt unfastened from the monotony and consist of the satisfaction of being alive.

Beyond the physical exertion, walking nurtures a profound thoughts-frame connection. As we synchronize our breath with every stride, we emerge as attuned to the rhythm of our our bodies. The constant beat of our hearts echoes in harmony with our footsteps, instilling a experience of balance and attention.

Running gives an avenue for meditation in motion, a sanctuary wherein we're capable of quiet our minds and find readability amidst the chaos of every day lifestyles. The endorphins released all through a run create a euphoric sensation, fostering a first-rate kingdom of thoughts and reducing pressure and tension.

Running is a powerful trainer, revealing our inner electricity and resilience. The moments whilst we push beyond our perceived limits and discover that we're able to greater than we imagined are transformative. As we conquer distances and stressful situations, we faucet into an unyielding wellspring of power of thoughts.

Through walking, we confront adversity and learn how to encompass discomfort as a stepping stone within the path of increase. The discipline and willpower required to enhance our walking capabilities increase past the trails and streets, shaping our individual and improving our capability to face existence's obstacles with grace and courage.

The Social Connection

While strolling regularly starts offevolved as a solitary pursuit, it has a excellent ability to forge connections with others. Running groups and golf equipment offer a enjoy of belonging and camaraderie. Shared research, mutual assist, and shared victories create bonds that increase past the finish line.

In institution runs and races, we come to be a part of something more than ourselves. The collective strength and encouragement of fellow runners inspire us to reach new heights and push thru moments of fatigue or doubt. Through going for walks, we find out our tribe, a supportive network that celebrates our accomplishments and shares in our satisfaction.

Running gives endless opportunities for success, from completing our first 5K race to conquering a hard marathon. Each milestone is a testomony to our perseverance and self-discipline. Crossing a cease line, no matter the gap, instills a profound experience of success that transcends into exceptional factors of our lives.

Running teaches us that fulfillment isn't measured actually via way of using winning races but via the journey and the increase we revel in along the way. Every step taken, each hill conquered, and every give up line crossed turns into a testomony to our spirit of resilience and our capability for achievement.

Running has a very particular manner of recuperation the mind, body, and soul. The repetitive motion of walking becomes a calming balm for the mind, helping to ease anxiety and despair. The bodily blessings of running, together with stepped forward cardiovascular fitness and strengthened muscular tissues, make a contribution to conventional properly-being.

Moreover, taking walks offers us an possibility to connect with our emotions. It allows us to approach our mind and feelings, imparting a cathartic release that opens the door to emotional restoration and self-discovery.

In a world filled with distractions, taking walks gives a treasured present—the present of living within the present 2d. As we lace up our shoes and take that first step, we launch the burdens of the beyond and the troubles of the destiny.

With each stride, we turn out to be acutely privy to the sensations of the winning—the feel of the ground under our ft, the rhythm of our breath, and the points of interest and sounds that surround us. Running becomes a moving meditation, a adventure into mindfulness in which we learn how to take pleasure in every 2nd actually.

Running permits us to shed the masks we located on in our every day lives and embrace our actual selves. In the solitude of a run, we discover an possibility for introspection, wherein we can be honest with ourselves and be aware of the whispers of our hearts.

Running becomes a canvas for self-expression, wherein we can be real and unapologetically ourselves. It's now not about competing with others however about difficult ourselves and turning into the satisfactory version of who we're.

The satisfaction of on foot goes past the physical act; it embodies a profound connection with ourselves and the sector round us. In the pursuit of freedom, we discover the strength interior, the camaraderie of like-minded souls, and the recuperation power of a transferring meditation.

As we lace up our shoes and step onto the open road, we embark on a journey of self-discovery, personal boom, and unwavering joy. Running will become a testomony to our resilience, a celebration of our achievements, and a reminder that the high-quality freedom lies in embracing the existing 2d and being real to ourselves. The delight of walking is an extended-lasting gift that beckons us to embark on this transformative adventure of movement, freedom, and self-discovery.

Chapter 12: Preparing For the Journey

As you step into the arena of walking, you embark on a transformative adventure of self-discovery and growth. To make sure a a hit and exciting enjoy, proper education is essential. In this financial ruin, we explore crucial guidelines and guidance for amateur runners, protective subjects which consist of putting sensible desires, establishing a robust schooling routine, records the importance of rest and recuperation, and locating motivation to hold shifting in advance.

As a newbie runner, it is vital to set sensible and potential goals. Setting the bar too immoderate can motive frustration and disappointment, at the identical time as modest and plausible goals assemble a sturdy basis for future growth.

Begin with the resource of knowledge your cutting-edge fitness level and setting incremental dreams. For example, reason to run for a specific duration or distance, progressively developing it through the years.

Celebrate every milestone you gain, irrespective of how small, as each breakthrough is a testament in your development.

A structured education normal is essential for improvement and harm prevention. Consistency is fundamental, so create a time desk that fits your way of existence and commitments.

Start with a possible amount of on foot days regular with week, permitting your body time to adapt and get higher. As you gain confidence and stamina, step by step growth the frequency and depth of your runs. Incorporate go-training and rest days into your everyday to preserve balance and reduce the threat of overuse injuries.

Investing in an exquisite pair of running footwear is one of the most important alternatives you can make as a beginner runner. Ill-fitting or beside the issue shoes can result in pain, pain, and damage.

Visit a distinctiveness on foot store in which experts can observe your gait and recommend footwear that offer the proper useful resource and cushioning in your foot kind. Properly turning into footwear will decorate your on foot revel in and decrease the chance of accidents.

A proper warmth-up and cool-down habitual are important additives of your on foot exercising. Warming up permits put together your body for the physical goals of going for walks, decreasing the threat of harm and enhancing general performance.

Before every run, engage in dynamic stretching physical sports and moderate jogging to elevate your coronary heart fee and increase blood drift for your muscle tissues. After your run, perform static stretches to improve flexibility and promote recovery.

Paying interest on your on foot shape is vital for efficiency and harm prevention. As a beginner, popularity on preserving an upright posture, attractive your center, and landing with a midfoot strike.

Avoid overstriding, as this can placed useless stress in your joints. Instead, reason for a cadence of round one hundred seventy-one hundred and eighty steps consistent with minute to decorate jogging performance.

Listening on your frame is crucial as you embark to your strolling journey. Pay interest to any symptoms of ache or pain and cope with them at once. It's ordinary to revel in a few muscle ache as you start jogging, but persistent pain or soreness may also want to indicate an damage.

Allow for accurate enough rest and healing amongst runs, mainly as your frame adapts to the today's needs of on foot. Rest is a important thing of your training, as it allows your muscle businesses to restore and extend stronger.

Proper hydration and vitamins are fundamental for fueling your runs and assisting in post-run restoration. Stay hydrated all through the day, and take into account carrying water with you sooner or later of your runs, specially in warmer weather.

Prioritize a balanced weight loss plan that consists of a mixture of carbohydrates, proteins, and healthful fats to aid your energy dreams. Fuel up earlier than longer runs and refuel with a put up-run snack or meal to top off glycogen stores and useful useful resource in muscle recuperation.

Running organizations can offer valuable help and camaraderie for newbie runners. Joining a community walking membership or participating in group runs may be motivating and frightening.

Running with others will can help you live responsible in your schooling everyday, percentage reviews, and gain treasured recommendation from extra professional runners. It's an opportunity to hook up with like-minded folks that percentage your passion for strolling.

As a amateur runner, you may come upon mental boundaries that venture your development. Self-doubt, worry of failure, or evaluating yourself to others can avoid your increase.

Remember that taking walks is a personal journey, and every runner's route is specific. Embrace the device, have an extraordinary time your achievements, and be type to yourself throughout difficult instances. Develop a fantastic mind-set and hobby at the pleasure of improvement and the texture of achievement each step brings.

Maintaining motivation as a amateur runner is essential for extended-time period achievement. Draw notion from diverse belongings, which incorporates reading books or articles approximately walking, following social media debts of professional runners, or looking documentaries approximately inspirational athletes.

Setting brief-time period and lengthy-time period goals can also fuel your motivation. Sign up for a race or task yourself to build up particular milestones to hold your enthusiasm alive.

As a amateur runner, embracing proper education and a awesome mind-set is important for a a success and amusing strolling journey. Setting realistic goals, setting up a training habitual, wearing appropriate on foot shoes, and listening to your body are foundational factors to keep in mind.

Chapter 13: Techniques to Improve Running Form

Running form is the spine of green and damage-loose strolling. As you development to your running adventure, honing your taking walks method turns into an increasing number of critical. In this bankruptcy, we delve into the intricacies of taking walks shape, find out common mistakes to keep away from, and provide realistic strategies to help you discover your stride and optimize your strolling mechanics.

Running shape refers back to the way you glide your body on the equal time as strolling. It includes the coordination of various body elements, which includes the arms, legs, torso, and head, to make sure green earlier motion.

The fundamentals of proper taking walks shape encompass:

1. Upright posture: Maintain a tall and upright posture to maximize lung ability and permit for inexperienced respiratory.

2. Arm swing: Your hands should swing manifestly at your aspects, bent at approximately ninety stages. Avoid crossing your hands during your frame, as it can waste electricity.

3. Relaxed shoulders: Keep your shoulders snug and keep away from tensing them, as anxiety could have an impact on your arm swing and standard shape.

four. Midfoot strike: Aim to land at the middle of your foot with each step, as this lets in distribute impact forces and decreases the threat of accidents.

five. Cadence: Strive for a cadence (steps in line with minute) of round a hundred and seventy-180, as a higher cadence is related to decreased effect forces and advanced strolling performance.

Common Running Form Mistakes

Identifying and correcting not unusual walking form mistakes is crucial for boosting your overall normal overall performance and reducing the chance of accidents. Some commonplace mistakes to take a look at out for embody:

1. Heel hanging: Landing for your heels with each step can purpose immoderate effect forces on your joints. Focus on touchdown at the midfoot or forefoot as an possibility.

2. Overstriding: Taking overly lengthy strides can cause braking forces and inefficient ahead motion. Aim for shorter, faster strides to enhance walking normal performance.

three. Hunching over: Poor posture, together with hunching over on the waist, can restrict respiratory and restriction your walking average performance. Keep your lower back immediately and shoulders snug.

four. Clenched fists: Tensing your fists while on foot can make a contribution to not unusual muscle tension. Keep your palms relaxed, alongside facet your fingers lightly curled.

5. Uneven arm swing: A lack of coordination in your arm swing could have an impact on your stability and large walking overall performance. Focus on keeping a herbal and symmetrical arm swing.

Techniques to Improve Running Form

Improving your running form is a sluggish approach that requires recognition, workout, and endurance. Here are a few techniques to help you discover your stride and decorate your on foot mechanics:

1. Video evaluation: Record yourself walking from numerous angles to have a examine your shape objectively. Analyze your posture, foot strike, arm swing, and cadence. Consider in search of feedback from a walking coach or skilled runner to understand areas for improvement.

2. Running drills: Incorporate taking walks drills into your schooling normal to beautify precise elements of your form. Drills along with excessive knees, butt kicks, and strides

can enhance cadence, stride length, and strolling monetary machine.

three. Focus on cadence: Strive to growth your cadence to the closing shape of 100 and seventy-one hundred and eighty steps in step with minute. Use a metronome app or strolling watch with a cadence feature to help you stay on the right track.

4. Core strengthening bodily activities: A sturdy middle is crucial for retaining right going for walks posture and balance. Include center strengthening physical video games, which incorporates planks and Russian twists, in your pass-education routine.

5. Run with a pal or organization: Running with others can offer instant remarks on your shape and offer motivation to hold properly method. Additionally, organization runs can introduce you to expert runners who can proportion treasured suggestions.

6. Mindful jogging: Practice aware taking walks by way of manner of focusing to your

shape, respiratory, and the sensations of your body. Regularly test in along with your posture, arm swing, and foot strike to maintain correct shape at some point of your run.

7. Gradual modifications: Making modifications in your walking form takes time. Avoid in search of to enforce all adjustments straight away. Instead, popularity on one element at a time, often incorporating it into your strolling habitual.

The Benefits of Improved Running Form

Investing time and effort in enhancing your going for walks form yields numerous benefits:

1. Injury prevention: Proper on foot form reduces the chance of commonplace taking walks accidents, which include shin splints, knee pain, and strain fractures.

2. Running overall performance: Optimal shape lets in you to use a lot less energy at the same time as on foot, developing your

staying power and standard taking walks overall performance.

three. Performance improvement: Improved form can bring about quicker race instances and advanced going for walks speed.

four. Enhanced amusement: Running with specific shape reduces pain and fatigue, allowing you to experience your runs to the fullest.

Finding your stride and perfecting your going for walks shape is an ongoing journey that requires self-control and exercising. Understanding the fundamentals of strolling shape, figuring out and correcting commonplace errors, and incorporating strategies to enhance your form will contribute to your growth as a runner.

With staying power and staying power, you can witness improvements to your universal performance, staying electricity, and average leisure of walking. As you refine your jogging shape, undergo in thoughts that each runner's shape is unique, and what subjects most is locating a fashion that works excellent for you.

By specializing in right walking mechanics, you lose up the functionality for entire lifestyles of damage-unfastened on foot, the satisfaction of pushing your obstacles, and the profound enjoy of fulfillment that comes from locating your stride on

Chapter 14: Nutrition for Peak Performance

Nutrition plays a essential function in helping your strolling common normal overall performance and trendy nicely-being. As a runner, your body requires the right stability of vitamins to gasoline your runs, useful resource in healing, and optimize your education efforts. In this bankruptcy, we find out the importance of vitamins for runners, delve into the vital detail nutrients desired for pinnacle basic performance, and offer sensible pointers at the manner to create a nicely-rounded nutrients plan to assist your strolling adventure.

The Role of Nutrition in Running

Proper vitamins is the cornerstone of a fulfillment taking walks. It offers the vital fuel to power your muscular tissues, keep electricity ranges, and manual maximum dependable traditional normal overall performance at some stage in training and races.

As a runner, your body undergoes accelerated bodily stress and energy expenditure. Ensuring you provide your frame with the right vitamins earlier than, in some unspecified time in the future of, and after your runs ought to make a huge distinction for your typical basic performance, endurance, and healing.

Key Nutrients for Runners

1. Carbohydrates: Carbohydrates are the primary deliver of strength for runners. They are damaged down into glucose, it is used as gasoline for muscles at some point of on foot. Complex carbohydrates, which include whole grains, fruits, and greens, offer sustained power, on the equal time as simple carbohydrates, like honey or sports sports beverages, can be useful for brief strength in the direction of lengthy runs or races.

2. Protein: Protein is vital for muscle restore and recovery. As a runner, you require slightly extra protein to guide your education efforts. Incorporate lean resources of protein, on the

facet of chook, fish, beans, tofu, and dairy merchandise, into your food and snacks.

three. Fats: Healthy fats, which includes those placed in avocados, nuts, seeds, and olive oil, provide a focused supply of electricity and resource numerous bodily functions. While carbohydrates are the number one fuel all through runs, fat play a crucial characteristic in longer staying power sports activities and retaining average health.

four. Hydration: Staying hydrated is important for runners to preserve maximum useful fashionable overall performance and prevent dehydration. Drink lots of water at some degree in the day, and hold in thoughts inclusive of electrolyte-rich liquids inside the direction of longer runs or in hot weather.

Creating a Nutrition Plan for Running

1. Pre-Run Nutrition: Before a run, intention for a balanced meal containing carbohydrates, protein, and a small amount of healthful fats. This meal ought to be

consumed as a minimum 1 to two hours in advance than your run to allow for digestion. If you're going for a shorter, easy run, a slight snack, including a banana or an electricity bar, may additionally additionally suffice.

2. During-Run Nutrition: For runs lasting longer than an hour, consider fueling with carbohydrates to preserve electricity degrees. Options embody strength gels, sports sports liquids, or without troubles digestible snacks like raisins or electricity chews.

3. Post-Run Nutrition: After a run, reputation on replenishing your glycogen stores and assisting in muscle recuperation. A combination of carbohydrates and protein is proper for a submit-run meal or snack. Chocolate milk, a turkey sandwich, or a smoothie with quit end result and Greek yogurt are exceptional options.

four. Hydration: Proper hydration is critical for best standard standard performance. Drink water in the course of the day and reason to drink earlier than, inside the path of, and after your runs. Pay interest in your frame's thirst cues and undergo in thoughts weighing your self earlier than and after longer runs to gauge fluid loss.

five. Nutrient Timing: Consider timing your meals and snacks strategically. Consuming a balanced meal with carbohydrates and protein internal 1/2-hour to an hour after a difficult workout can optimize restoration and muscle repair.

6. Listen to Your Body: Every runner's dietary goals are specific. Pay interest to how your frame responds to extremely good factors and alter your vitamins plan hence. Consulting with a registered dietitian who specializes in sports sports sports vitamins may be beneficial in tailoring a plan that suits your person wishes and dreams.

The Importance of Balanced Meals

A balanced eating regimen is important for runners, as it gives a massive type of vitamins wished for common health and nicely-being.

Focus on developing food that embody lots of culmination, veggies, entire grains, lean proteins, and wholesome fats.

Incorporate a rainbow of colourful fruits and veggies into your weight loss plan, as they offer a huge range of vitamins, minerals, and antioxidants. Whole grains, inclusive of quinoa, brown rice, and oats, offer sustained energy and critical vitamins.

Lean assets of protein, which encompass fowl, turkey, fish, beans, lentils, and tofu, assist muscle restore and recuperation. Healthy fats from avocados, nuts, seeds, and olive oil are critical for mobile health and also can make contributions to satiety throughout longer runs.

While a balanced diet ought to offer maximum of the nutrients you want as a runner, high first-class supplements also can benefit your overall performance and normal health. It's critical to are searching for advice from a healthcare professional or registered dietitian earlier than along with any nutritional supplements on your nutrients plan.

Common nutritional supplements for runners embody:

1. Electrolytes: Electrolyte supplements or sports activities liquids can help maintain proper fluid stability and prevent dehydration for the duration of lengthy runs or in heat situations.

2. Iron: Female runners, mainly, can also moreover gain from iron nutritional supplements if they will be prone to iron deficiency because of heavy menstrual durations or inadequate iron consumption.

three. Vitamin D: If you've got got had been given constrained sun exposure or live in a vicinity with low sunlight, food plan D supplementation can be useful for bone health and immune function.

4. Omega-three Fatty

Chapter 15: Building Mental Resilience in Running

Running isn't always only a bodily pursuit; it's also a mental journey that annoying conditions our inner energy and resilience. As a runner, you may always come across boundaries, self-doubt, and moments of conflict. In this financial disaster, we find out the significance of building intellectual resilience in going for walks, understanding the psychological elements of the game, and providing practical strategies to conquer disturbing conditions and domesticate a robust and superb mind-set.

Running is a deeply personal and introspective hobby. Beyond the physical wishes, it requires intellectual fortitude and the functionality to confront and overcome mental barriers.

The mental components of taking walks encompass:

1. Self-Motivation: Running often includes solitary schooling schooling and prolonged

runs in which self-motivation becomes paramount. The ability to stay centered, set dreams, and preserve enthusiasm at some point of your education is vital.

2. Goal Setting: Setting sensible and good sized desires is a important a part of the jogging adventure. Whether it's completing your first 5K race, enhancing your race time, or conquering a marathon, well-defined dreams provide a revel in of cause and route.

3. Mental Toughness: Developing highbrow durability permits you to push via demanding situations, pain, and fatigue throughout runs and races. It entails the potential to stay resilient, focused, and high-quality, even in negative conditions.

4. Mindfulness: Running can function a shape of moving meditation, in which you domesticate mindfulness with the aid of using being absolutely gift within the 2d, looking your mind and sensations with out judgment.

five. Managing Pre-Race Nerves: Pre-race nerves are not unusual among runners. Learning to control race-day tension and nerves is critical to preserving interest and confidence.

Practical Strategies for Building Mental Resilience

1. Embrace Positive Self-Talk: Cultivate a terrific inner speak in some unspecified time in the future of your runs and schooling. Replace self-doubt and poor mind with encouraging and supportive affirmations. Remind yourself of your beyond achievements and the improvement you have made.

2. Break Down Goals: Rather than feeling overwhelmed thru prolonged-term goals, ruin them down into smaller, capacity milestones. Celebrate every milestone reached, as they may be stepping stones within the direction of your remaining intention.

three. Visualization: Visualization is a effective tool for building mental resilience. Before races or difficult runs, near your eyes and vividly consider yourself crossing the give up line with electricity and determination.

4. Focus on the Process: Instead of obsessing over the final outcomes, awareness at the way of jogging itself. Concentrate on your breath, your shape, and the rhythm of your footsteps. This mindfulness permits you to live gift and perform at your pleasant.

five. Reframe Challenges: Shift your angle on worrying conditions and setbacks. Rather than viewing them as disasters, see them as opportunities for boom and mastering. Every obstacle you conquer makes you stronger and further resilient.

6. Practice Mental Toughness: Embrace hard runs and exercising exercises as opportunities to increase intellectual durability. When managing fatigue or soreness, remind yourself which you have the intellectual energy to push via.

7. Establish a Mantra: Create a private mantra that resonates with you. Repeat it inside the direction of hard moments to live targeted and recommended. Your mantra may be as easy as "I am robust" or "I can try this."

eight. Learn from Setbacks: Accept that setbacks are a herbal a part of the on foot adventure. Use them as treasured learning reports, allowing you to refine your method and grow as a runner.

nine. Surround Yourself with Positive Influences: Seek out a supportive taking walks network or education companions who can offer encouragement and camaraderie. Sharing tales and dreams with like-minded humans can be uplifting and upsetting.

10. Practice Gratitude: Cultivate a attitude of gratitude for the possibility to run and the development you have made. Gratitude shifts your interest from what you lack to what you have, fostering a first-rate and resilient mind-set.

Overcoming Pre-Race Nerves

Pre-race nerves are a not unusual enjoy for runners of all tiers. Managing the ones nerves can drastically impact your race-day universal overall performance. Here are some strategies to conquer pre-race jitters:

1. Familiarize Yourself with the Course: Study the race route and visualize yourself running it successfully. Knowing what to expect can reduce tension on race day.

2. Develop a Race-Day Routine: Establish a familiar race-day ordinary that includes pre-race meals, heat-up wearing sports, and highbrow schooling. Following a routine can create a experience of familiarity and control.

three. Focus on What You Can Control: Accept that a few factors, which include weather conditions or the overall overall performance of different runners, are beyond your manage. Concentrate on what you can manipulate, consisting of your thoughts-set and race method.

4. Breathe and Relax: Practice deep respiratory strategies to calm your nerves. Before the race, find out a quiet spot to respire deeply and relax your frame.

5. Visualization: Use visualization to mentally rehearse your race, together with precise conditions and the manner you can reply to them. Imagine yourself handling challenges with self guarantee and determination.

6. Trust Your Training: Remember the hours of education you've got established to put together for the race. Trust for your abilities and the artwork you have executed to get to the start line.

7. Focus at the Experience: Shift your popularity from the very last consequences to the enjoy of racing. Embrace the pride of strolling and the camaraderie of the event.

As a runner, building highbrow resilience is as essential as bodily schooling. It lets in you to triumph over demanding situations, get higher from setbacks, and perform at your exceptional, even in the face of adversity.

Resilience is a skill that extends beyond taking walks, reaping benefits numerous areas of your lifestyles. It complements your functionality to address strain, adapt to change, and maintain a splendid outlook.

By incorporating sensible strategies for constructing highbrow resilience, you liberate the potential for increase, self-discovery, and private achievement on your strolling adventure. Embrace the stressful situations, be given as right with to your talents, and domesticate a attitude that celebrates the adventure of walking as masses because the vacation spot. In doing so, you switch out to be a more potent

Strategies for Personal Growth

Goal placing is a powerful device for personal boom and success in taking walks. Whether you are a novice or an professional runner, having easy and massive goals offers route and motive in your schooling and racing endeavors. In this economic catastrophe, we find out the art work of putting effective on foot desires, developing a properly-set up plan to acquire them, and the transformative effect of reason attainment in your on foot adventure.

Setting desires in on foot goes past honestly completing a race or attaining a specific time. Goals provide a roadmap in your taking walks adventure, guiding your efforts, and assisting you stay advocated and focused.

The advantages of intention placing in running embody:

1. Focus and Direction: Goals offer you with a clean reputation and path on your education and races. They help you prioritize your efforts and avoid distractions.

2. Motivation: Meaningful goals serve as a powerful supply of motivation, pushing you to constantly art work in the direction of your targets.

3. Measuring Progress: Goals offer benchmarks for measuring your development and boom as a runner. They assist you to song improvements over the years.

4. Overcoming Plateaus: Setting tough dreams assist you to spoil via plateaus and push past your consolation place.

5. Building Confidence: Achieving desires builds self assurance and self-notion, empowering you to set even greater ambitious dreams.

Types of Running Goals

When putting taking walks dreams, bear in mind the specific forms of objectives you may pursue:

1. Performance Goals: These dreams hobby on carrying out precise race instances, non-public bests, or ratings in competitions.

2. Endurance Goals: Endurance dreams contain completing longer distance races, in

conjunction with a half marathon, marathon, or ultramarathon.

three. Skill Goals: Skill desires attention on enhancing precise factors of your taking walks method, along side form, cadence, or hill strolling.

four. Consistency Goals: Consistency desires contain retaining a regular education time desk, committing to a certain wide variety of weekly runs, or strolling for a tough and rapid kind of days in step with month.

five. Race Goals: These desires revolve round taking part particularly races or events, either to enjoy the environment or venture your self with particular conditions.

Creating SMART Goals

Effective purpose putting includes growing SMART dreams—dreams which is probably Specific, Measurable, Achievable, Relevant, and Time-certain. Follow those pointers to boom your SMART going for walks dreams:

1. Specific: Clearly outline your purpose. Specify what you need to advantage and why it is critical to you. For instance, in region of pronouncing, "I want to run quicker," specify, "I want to decorate my 10K race time via 2 mins."

2. Measurable: Set concrete standards to degree your development and fulfillment. Use quantifiable metrics, which encompass race instances or distances, to music your basic performance.

three. Achievable: Make positive your desires are practical and viable. While it's miles essential to task yourself, placing unrealistic goals may also moreover bring about frustration and burnout.

4. Relevant: Ensure your goals align together along with your running aspirations and popular lifestyles dreams. Ask yourself how mission the aim will make contributions on your non-public growth and fulfilment as a runner.

5. Time-positive: Set a closing date or goal date for conducting your cause. A time-certain aim gives a enjoy of urgency and helps you live centered on your schooling.

Creating a Goal-Setting Plan

1. Reflect on Your Running Journey: Take time to mirror in your past walking reviews and accomplishments. Identify regions in which you have had been given excelled and areas wherein you need to improve.

2. Set Short-Term and Long-Term Goals: Develop each brief-term and prolonged-term desires. Short-time period dreams preserve you influenced and offer stepping stones toward your final goals.

3. Prioritize Your Goals: If you have were given a couple of goals, prioritize them based totally on their significance and feasibility. Focusing on some key dreams at a time permits you to direct your energy greater efficaciously.

4. Break Goals into Actionable Steps: Break down your desires into smaller, actionable steps. This technique makes them an awful lot less overwhelming and allows you create a smooth route to fulfillment.

five. Seek Support and Accountability: Share your goals with buddies, family, or strolling partners. Having a guide device and a person to hold you accountable can be pretty motivating.

6. Monitor Your Progress: Regularly music your development towards your desires. Celebrate your achievements and regulate your approach if critical.

Overcoming Obstacles and Adjusting Goals

As with any adventure, your going for walks goals may additionally come upon obstacles and stressful situations along the way. Be organized to comply and alter your goals as wanted. Factors collectively with harm, changes in existence activities, or surprising sports may additionally require revising your timeline or expectations.

When dealing with setbacks, endure in thoughts that resilience is a essential problem of goal pursuit. Embrace traumatic situations as opportunities to investigate and develop, and use them to reinforce your willpower and determination to your dreams.

When adjusting your dreams, be sensible approximately what is workable inside the given situations. Embrace flexibility and recognize that setbacks are a natural part of the tool. With each adjustment, reaffirm your dedication to your walking journey and the private boom it offers.

Achieving your taking walks desires is a transformative experience that extends past the place of walking. The adventure of setting and working towards your dreams instills place, resilience, and self-notion.

Chapter 16: Embracing the Running Community and Its Impact

Running is not definitely an individual pursuit; it's miles a network that brings human beings collectively from all walks of lifestyles, united thru a shared passion for the sport. In this economic catastrophe, we delve into the significance of the taking walks network, the assist and camaraderie it gives, and the transformative effect it could must your jogging journey.

At its middle, running is a solo interest, but the taking walks community gives a brand new period to the game. Whether you're a amateur or an experienced runner, becoming a member of the walking community can offer useful guide, notion, and a revel in of belonging.

1. Camaraderie: Running with others fosters a experience of camaraderie that can make the hardest of runs experience much less complex. The shared enjoy of overcoming disturbing conditions and celebrating

achievements creates a very particular bond amongst runners.

2. Motivation: Surrounding yourself with like-minded folks that are committed to their on foot dreams may be alternatively motivating. The encouragement and duty from the community push you to be regular and strive for improvement.

three. Learning and Sharing: The taking walks community is a treasure trove of knowledge and experience. Runners of all degrees percentage insights, hints, and education strategies, assisting each awesome develop and evolve as athletes.

4. Inclusivity: The strolling network embraces variety and inclusivity, welcoming runners of each age, backgrounds, and competencies. It's an area wherein everybody is united with the useful resource of using their love for strolling, irrespective of their tempo or distance.

five. Social Support: The going for walks community gives a network of assist past the game itself. Many lifelong friendships are fashioned in the direction of training instructions, races, and jogging sports.

Ways to Engage with the Running Community

1. Join a Running Club: Local walking golf equipment are a exceptional way to connect with extraordinary runners for your vicinity. Look for golf equipment that align along with your goals and hobbies, whether or not or now not it's far casual strolling, aggressive racing, or path running.

2. Participate in Group Runs: Many walking golf equipment arrange normal institution runs, which offer a enjoy of shape and social engagement for your education ordinary. These runs regularly variety in distance and tempo, accommodating runners of numerous talents.

3. Volunteer at Races: Volunteering at races is an top notch way to immerse your self in the

walking network. You can assist with race business enterprise, useful useful resource stations, or cheering on fellow runners.

4. Attend Running Events: Participate in close by going for walks sports activities, which includes charity races, a laugh runs, or themed runs. These occasions provide a colorful surroundings and the possibility to fulfill and connect with extremely good runners.

5. Online Running Communities: Engage with the jogging network thru on line systems and social media. Online boards, taking walks companies on social media, and strolling apps can offer a virtual vicinity for connecting with other runners global.

The resource and encouragement from the strolling network should have a profound effect on your taking walks journey and easy properly-being.

1. Increased Motivation: Being part of a supportive community conjures up you to

stay consistent along side your education and push yourself to gain your dreams.

2. Accountability: When you apprehend others are relying on you, it motivates you to expose up for institution runs and schooling training, even on days while you can feel much less stimulated.

3. Overcoming Challenges: The collective manual of the strolling network lets in you conquer boundaries and navigate thru moments of self-doubt or setbacks.

4. Learning and Growth: Engaging with other runners exposes you to severa perspectives and education techniques, fostering non-stop mastering and personal increase.

5. Celebration of Success: The on foot community is brief to have a good time each unique's successes, every huge and small, developing a powerful and uplifting environment.

Running for a Cause - Charity and Social Impact

Running furthermore offers an road for creating a effective social impact. Many runners take part in charity races and fundraising activities, the usage of their ardour for taking walks to help numerous reasons.

1. Charity Races: Charity races increase price range and interest for nonprofit agencies and social motives. By taking part in the ones races, you're making a contribution to a larger social mission on the equal time as pursuing your strolling goals.

2. Personal Fundraising: Some runners take their willpower a step in addition by means of manner of starting personal fundraising campaigns for reasons they deeply care about. This strive amplifies the effect of their strolling journey beyond their personal achievements.

three. Community Engagement: The jogging network often comes together to useful resource community obligations and network outreach programs. These efforts beautify the bonds in the community and amplify their awesome effect to the wider society.

The Transformative Impact of the Running Community

Beyond the physical and highbrow advantages of walking, the walking community has the strength to impact profound versions in the lives of its individuals.

1. Confidence and Belonging: Being a part of a supportive community instills a experience of self guarantee and belonging. It empowers you to include your identity as a runner and a treasured member of the community.

2. Social Connection: The going for walks community expands your social circle, imparting opportunities to fulfill people from particular backgrounds and cultures. This enriches your lifestyles and broadens your horizons.

three. Overcoming Barriers: The revel in of camaraderie in the network allows you overcome boundaries you can have previously perceived as insurmountable.

four. Inspiration and Role Models: In the strolling community, you encounter runners who've completed first-rate feats. Their memories of willpower and resilience encourage you to push past your limits and dream big.

5. Lifelong Friendships: Many runners form lifelong friendships via the network. These friendships are built on shared testimonies, mutual beneficial resource, and a commonplace passion for going for walks.

Giving Back to the Running Community

As you enjoy the transformative effect of the on foot community, undergo in thoughts giving once more and being an active player in assisting others on their taking walks journey.

1. Encourage New Runners: Support new runners as they take their first steps into the game. Offer advice, percentage your opinions, and be a supply of encouragement.

2. Volunteer and Coach: Volunteer at races or hold in thoughts turning into a on foot train or mentor. Your know-how and steering can honestly have an impact at the development of various runners.

three. Share Knowledge and Inspiration: Share your information and on foot evaluations through on-line systems, blogs, or social media. Your insights and recollections can encourage and encourage others.

The strolling network is a colourful and empowering community of those who percent a common love for the sport. Embracing the walking community can increase the joy and success you revel in from running, providing assist, motivation, and a experience of belonging.

Through the electricity of connection, the running community fosters resilience, private boom, and a determination to growing a pleasant social effect. Engaging with the network enriches your taking walks adventure, introduces you to lifelong friendships, and broadens your horizons.

As you immerse yourself within the walking network, cherish the collective spirit that unites runners international. Celebrate your successes, help others of their pursuits, and encompass the transformative impact of the strolling community on your adventure as a runner and as part of a few components plenty greater than yourself.

Chapter 17: The Art of Recovery

In the pursuit of taking walks dreams, it is simple to get stuck up in the pleasure of training, racing, and accomplishing new milestones. However, one important element that regularly gets overlooked is recuperation. Recovery is the crucial element to not only stopping injuries but moreover maximizing performance and traditional nicely-being. In this chapter, we discover the artwork of recovery, statistics its importance, and providing sensible strategies to nurture your body and mind for most green traditional typical overall performance and durability in taking walks.

Recovery is the technique of allowing your body to heal and adapt after the bodily strain of running. It is at a few level inside the restoration segment that your muscular tissues restore and increase more potent, and your cardiovascular system improves its overall performance.

The significance of recovery in strolling can be summarized as follows:

1. Injury Prevention: Proper healing reduces the hazard of overuse accidents, along with stress fractures, tendinitis, and muscle traces. Giving your body adequate time to rest and get better is vital for stopping accidents as a consequence of overtraining.

2. Performance Enhancement: Effective recovery leads to advanced overall performance. When you permit your body to get higher honestly among workout workouts, your muscles and strength systems grow to be greater efficient, fundamental to greater applicable walking generic usual performance.

3. Muscle Repair and Growth: During rest, your muscle mass undergo repair and boom, becoming more potent and additional resilient. This device is important for adapting to the wishes of schooling and achieving your running dreams.

4. Mental Well-being: Recovery isn't always quite an entire lot bodily relaxation; it also includes intellectual rejuvenation. Giving your thoughts time to decompress and loosen up is critical for retaining a satisfactory mind-set and avoiding burnout.

five. Sleep Quality: Recovery is cautiously associated with sleep awesome. A particular night time's sleep is crucial for bodily and intellectual recovery, and it plays a crucial function in typical overall performance and normal fitness.

Strategies for Effective Recovery

1. Listen to Your Body: Pay near interest to your body's signs. If you enjoy ache, fatigue, or uncommon pain, take it as a signal that you could want more rest or a lighter schooling load.

2. Adequate Sleep: Aim for 7-nine hours of first-rate sleep consistent with night time. Sleep is at the same time as your body undergoes most of its repair and

regeneration, making it a vital element of recovery.

3. Nutrition: Proper nutrients performs a primary function in recovery. Ensure you consume a balanced food plan wealthy in nutrients to help muscle repair and pinnacle off energy shops.

4. Hydration: Stay safely hydrated in some unspecified time in the future of the day. Proper hydration is crucial for optimizing physical ordinary overall performance and recuperation.

5. Active Recovery: Incorporate energetic restoration activities, collectively with gentle stretching, yoga, or slight pass-training, for your relaxation days. Active recuperation promotes blood waft to muscles and lets in with muscle discomfort.

6. Foam Rolling and Massage: Foam rolling can be useful in releasing muscle tension and improving flexibility. Consider getting a rub

down to relieve muscle pain and enhance recuperation.

7. Compression Garments: Some runners discover compression garments useful in decreasing muscle soreness and swelling placed up-run.

eight. Ice Baths: After intense exercise exercises or races, keep in mind taking ice baths to reduce contamination and boost up muscle restoration.

nine. Rest Days: Include scheduled rest days for your training plan. Rest days are virtually as vital as education days, allowing your body to get better and rebuild.

10. Cross-Training: Engage in bypass-training sports activities sports that complement strolling, which consist of swimming, cycling, or electricity education. Cross-education offers a damage from repetitive motions and may lessen the danger of overuse accidents.

The Role of Mental Recovery

Recovery is not just about bodily factors; mental restoration is in addition important. Running may be mentally worrying, and it is important to offer your thoughts time to relaxation and recharge.

1. Mindfulness and Meditation: Incorporate mindfulness and meditation practices into your routine. These practices assist reduce pressure, beautify attention, and promote mental readability.

2. Stress Management: Identify and manipulate assets of stress in your existence. Chronic strain can negatively impact your bodily and intellectual nicely-being, affecting your recuperation and performance.

3. Disconnect from Technology: Take breaks from monitors and digital devices, specially in advance than bedtime. Allow your self time to unwind and disconnect from the virtual international.

4. Visualization: Use visualization strategies to mentally rehearse a fulfillment runs and

races. Visualization can enhance self assurance and performance while it subjects most.

five. Enjoyment and Balance: Remember that strolling need to be fun and fun. Find a balance among schooling and special factors of your existence to prevent burnout.

Overcoming Barriers to Recovery

Despite knowledge the significance of healing, many runners warfare to position into impact effective recovery practices. Several boundaries can save you proper recovery, however reputation and proactive measures can help conquer them:

1. Time Constraints: Busy schedules and other commitments should make it difficult to prioritize recuperation. Plan your education agenda mindfully to consist of appropriate sufficient relaxation days and recovery sports.

2. Fear of Losing Fitness: Some runners fear that taking relaxation days or decreasing schooling depth will cause a loss of fitness. In

reality, recovery is vital for lengthy-term progress and damage prevention.

3. Lack of Knowledge: Some runners may be blind to the significance of healing or uncertain approximately the first rate healing practices. Educate yourself on restoration techniques and their benefits to optimize your schooling.

4. Overtraining: Pushing yourself too difficult without top enough rest can purpose overtraining, causing bodily and intellectual burnout. Be privy to your training load and the indicators your body is sending.

five. Social Pressure: The competitive nature of strolling and the selection to keep up with others can sometimes purpose neglecting recuperation. Remember that each runner's dreams are one-of-a-type, and what works for others may not be just proper for you.

The Transformative Impact of Prioritizing Recovery

By prioritizing recuperation, you lay the foundation for a a success and sustainable jogging adventure. Embracing the art of recuperation gives transformative benefits that make bigger past walking:

1. Enhanced Performance: Proper restoration optimizes your body's functionality to evolve to education, most important to advanced overall performance and faster development within the path of your going for walks desires.

2. Injury Prevention: Taking care of your body through recovery practices reduces the threat of accidents, allowing you to live regular in your education and racing.

3. Mental Clarity: Mental recovery enhances recognition, recognition, and general highbrow clarity, benefiting all regions of your existence.

4. Longevity in Running: Prioritizing recovery fosters a sustainable taking walks workout,

permitting you to revel in the game for years yet to come.

five. Joy and Fulfillment: Running turns into a supply of delight and fulfillment at the same time as you find out a stability among training, recovery, and various factors of your lifestyles.

Recovery is the cornerstone of a fulfillment and satisfying going for walks. By nurturing your frame and thoughts via powerful recuperation techniques, you maximize performance, save you injuries, and cultivate a sustainable taking walks exercise.

Embrace the paintings of healing as an imperative a part of your on foot journey. Prioritize rest, nutrients, and highbrow rejuvenation to unfastened up the transformative energy of recovery. As you integrate those practices into your education, you may discover that now not only does your strolling regular overall performance decorate, however your commonplace properly-being and enjoyment of the game increase to new heights. Remember, in the artwork of restoration, you find out the call of the sport to turning into a greater in form, happier, and extra resilient runner.

Embracing Adaptability - Navigating Change and Challenges in Running

As with any adventure in lifestyles, the route of a runner isn't always constantly smooth or predictable. Running, like existence, is filled with moments of exchange, demanding situations, and sudden conditions. In this financial disaster, we discover the importance of embracing adaptability in taking walks, knowledge the way to navigate through exchange, and building resilience to conquer demanding situations for your running journey.

The Nature of Adaptability in Running

Adaptability in strolling refers to the capability to modify, evolve, and respond effectively to changing instances. These adjustments can occur in numerous office work:

1. Physical Changes: Your body isn't always a static entity; it constantly evolves with education, age, and out of doors factors. Adapting to bodily adjustments is vital for keeping performance and stopping accidents.

2. Environmental Changes: Weather situations, terrain, and race settings can all vary notably. Adapting to as a minimum one-of-a-type environments is important for performing optimally in any situation.

three. Life Changes: Life sports, on the aspect of career transitions, circle of relatives obligations, or personal disturbing conditions, can effect your jogging ordinary. Embracing adaptability allows you to find out new strategies to contain jogging into your life.

four. Performance Fluctuations: Running standard performance may not normally progress linearly. There can be americaand downs, and embracing adaptability allows you navigate thru performance fluctuations.

Embracing adaptability isn't always quite a bargain reacting to exchange; it is about proactively making equipped yourself for the inevitable fluctuations in your walking adventure. Here's why adaptability topics in jogging:

1. Injury Prevention: Adapting your education utility to residence changes to your frame and health stages can save you overuse injuries and setbacks.

2. Continued Progress: Adaptability permits you to preserve making improvement even all through difficult times, making sure you stay heading inside the proper route on the side of your taking walks dreams.

three. Mental Resilience: Being open to trade and embracing adaptability fosters intellectual resilience, allowing you to stay outstanding and encouraged within the course of hard intervals.

four. Enjoyment of Running: Embracing adaptability permits you preserve a sense of delight and success in strolling, even supposing times are plenty less than ideal.

Practical Strategies for Embracing Adaptability

1. Listen to Your Body: Pay near interest in your body's signs and adjust your education therefore. If you revel in fatigued or enjoy pain, recall taking more relaxation or improving your carrying activities.

2. Flexibility in Training: Be flexible with your education time table. If existence sports activities or surprising events disrupt your deliberate exercise exercises, discover opportunity instances or adapt your education plan for that reason.

3. Cross-Training: Cross-schooling offers an possibility to differ your workout workout routines and supply specific muscles a smash. Embrace go-schooling sports activities that complement your strolling while imparting a change of tempo.

four. Adjust Goals: Be open to adjusting your strolling goals at the same time as wanted. Life sports or modifications in instances might also require you to recalibrate your dreams.

5. Mental Adaptability: Develop a mindset of adaptability and resilience. Cultivate an thoughts-set that embraces exchange and perspectives demanding conditions as possibilities for boom.

6. Seek Support: Surround yourself with a supportive network of buddies, circle of relatives, or taking walks partners who can provide encouragement and information in some unspecified time in the future of hard times.

Navigating Change in Running

Life is dynamic, and alternate is inevitable. When navigating trade in your strolling adventure, undergo in mind the subsequent techniques:

1. Gradual Adaptation: When making massive adjustments for your education recurring,

allow for sluggish model. Sudden adjustments can reason injuries or burnout.

2. Periodization: Embrace periodization for your schooling, which includes deliberate versions extensive and amount. Periodization permits your frame to comply to top notch schooling hundreds.

3. Seek Professional Guidance: If you come upon incredible bodily changes or traumatic conditions, bear in mind searching out steering from a train or healthcare professional.

four. Embrace Diversity: Incorporate a number of carrying occasions and terrains into your education. This range prepares you to deal with exceptional race situations and settings.

Building Resilience inside the Face of Challenges

Running, like lifestyles, will gift you with traumatic conditions and boundaries. Building resilience is crucial for navigating via hard times. Here's a way to assemble resilience in jogging:

1. Positive Mindset: Cultivate a powerful and wonderful outlook. Focus on what you could manage and adopt a "can-do" thoughts-set.

2. Learn from Setbacks: Instead of viewing setbacks as screw ups, see them as studying opportunities. Reflect on what you could beautify and use those tales to grow.

3. Set Realistic Expectations: Set manageable goals and recognize that improvement may not always be linear. Celebrate small victories and milestones along the way.

4. Self-Compassion: Be kind to your self and keep away from self-complaint. Understand that everyone faces demanding conditions, and it's miles ok to take time to regroup and refocus.

5. Visualize Success: Use visualization strategies to photo your self overcoming demanding situations and attaining your

strolling dreams. Visualization reinforces your perception for your talents.

Finding Joy within the Journey

Embracing adaptability and constructing resilience permits you to locate pleasure in the adventure of on foot. The demanding situations and modifications you come across grow to be opportunities for growth and self-discovery. Embrace the method, and don't forget that the adventure of running isn't just about the vacation spot however approximately the tales, relationships, and private increase you come upon alongside the way.

Adaptability is an essential ability for any runner on the lookout for long-term success and achievement in the game. Embracing adaptability permits you to navigate through modifications, overcome challenges, and construct resilience in your jogging adventure. Whether it's miles adjusting your schooling recurring, enhancing your goals, or embracing the fluctuations of overall performance, adaptability empowers you to thrive as a runner.

Find pleasure in the journey, encompass the modifications, and get pleasure from the memories that on foot offers. Embracing adaptability isn't always pretty plenty turning into a better runner; it's miles approximately turning into a more potent and additional resilient man or woman every on and rancid the road. In the face of trade and stressful conditions, do not forget that your adaptability and resilience are what is going to supply you through to new heights on your taking walks adventure.

Chapter 18: The Journey Continues

As you improvement for your on foot adventure, keeping extended-term motivation and passion becomes vital for persisted growth and enjoyment in the sport. The allure of walking regularly lies in the initial pride of placing dreams and engaging in milestones. However, maintaining enthusiasm and self-control through the years requires deliberate try and a deep connection to the essence of taking walks. In this chapter, we find out the keys to maintaining lengthy-term jogging motivation and ardour, so your journey stays a source of achievement and private boom.

Intrinsic motivation stems from internal elements inclusive of personal delight, leisure, and a enjoy of reason. Cultivating intrinsic motivation is vital for retaining prolonged-time period ardour in walking. Here's a manner to nurture intrinsic motivation:

1. Reflect on Your Why: Reconnect with the reasons you started out going for walks in the

first region. Reflect on how strolling makes you experience and the excessive incredible impact it has on your lifestyles.

2. Set Meaningful Goals: Set desires that align together with your values and aspirations. Meaningful goals supply reason and direction in your strolling journey.

three. Focus at the Process: Shift your attention from honestly very last consequences-based absolutely wants to playing the approach of on foot. Embrace the small victories, the pride of each run, and the increase you experience along the manner.

4. Celebrate Progress: Celebrate your development and achievements, regardless of how small. Acknowledging your efforts reinforces your motivation and builds confidence.

5. Embrace Challenges: View challenges as opportunities for boom in place of limitations. Embracing demanding situations fosters a

increase thoughts-set and resilience for your walking adventure.

Balancing Ambition and Enjoyment

Balancing ambition and entertainment is prime to sustaining prolonged-term ardour in on foot. While placing bold dreams is crucial, it's similarly vital to find out pride inside the day by day act of walking. Here's a manner to strike this balance:

1. Embrace Versatility: Vary your strolling routine to hold it clean and fun. Incorporate notable types of runs, explore new routes, and interact in occasional social runs with buddies or a walking commercial enterprise company.

2. Listen to Your Body: Pay attention to how your body feels and alter your training to keep away from burnout or overtraining. Embrace relaxation days and restoration sports activities to nurture every your body and thoughts.

3. Race for Fun: Participate in races truly for the enjoy and camaraderie, in desire to focusing mostly on private information. Race day may be a celebration of your adventure and the pleasure of on foot.

four. Incorporate Playfulness: Embrace a enjoy of playfulness in your jogging. Run with out a specific plan or tempo on occasion and permit your instincts guide you.

Building a Supportive Network

Having a supportive network is treasured for retaining prolonged-term motivation and ardour in strolling. Surround yourself with like-minded folks who percent your love for the sport. Here's a manner to assemble a supportive community:

1. Join a Running Club: Joining a community running club offers opportunities for organization runs, schooling schooling, and social sports. The camaraderie and help of fellow runners can be uplifting and inspiring.

2. Online Communities: Engage with on-line strolling agencies and social media groups. These digital regions permit you to hook up with runners from all around the global, exchange studies, and discover motivation.

three. Running Partners: Find a taking walks companion who shares your tempo and dreams. Running with a partner can offer mutual motivation, responsibility, and leisure.

four. Family Support: Share your strolling adventure together with your family, and incorporate them on your races and accomplishments. Their aid and encouragement may be a significant supply of motivation.

Fueling Your Passion

Fueling your passion for jogging consists of nurturing your mind, frame, and soul. Here are vital factors to keep in thoughts:

1. Mindfulness and Gratitude: Practice mindfulness at some point of your runs, staying present and appreciating the splendor

of every 2nd. Cultivate gratitude for the ability to run and the studies it brings.

2. Continuous Learning: Stay curious and constantly are trying to find opportunities to find out about going for walks, education techniques, and the stories of diverse runners.

3. Connect with Nature: Running in nature may be a religious revel in, fostering a deep connection with the area spherical you.

4. Inspiring Content: Read taking walks books, watch documentaries, or pay attention to podcasts about running. These belongings of concept can reignite your ardour for the game.

5. Setting Challenges: Set periodic traumatic situations to keep your on foot adventure interesting. This can embody attempting a modern-day race distance, jogging in a specific area, or exploring a path run.

Finding Balance with Other Aspects of Life

Maintaining balance amongst running and various factors of your existence is vital for retaining lengthy-term motivation and ardour. Here's the way to find this balance:

1. Time Management: Plan your training and walking sports around your particular commitments. Creating a time table that consists of all elements of your life can reduce strain and save you conflicts.

2. Prioritizing Rest: Embrace rest and recuperation as critical additives of your education. Rest permits you to recharge bodily and mentally, preventing burnout.

three. Family and Social Engagement: Balance your walking pastimes with first-rate time spent with own family and friends. Engaging in social sports activities past jogging enriches your existence and offers emotional help.

Embracing the Evolution of Running

Chapter 19: The Basics of Running

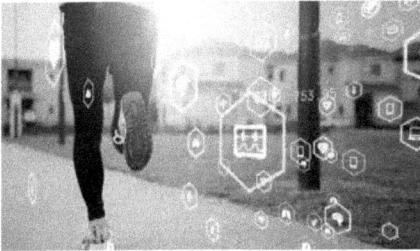

Running:

Running is a form of cardio workout that involves shifting hastily walking, usually at a tempo quicker than strolling. It is a famous and to be had bodily hobby that offers numerous health advantages, which encompass progressed cardiovascular health, weight manipulate, superior temper, and prolonged staying power. Running can range vast and period, from brief sprints to prolonged-distance marathons. It engages severa muscle businesses and is an effective manner to burn strength and stay match.

Fasting:

Fasting refers to the intentional abstention from meals or caloric consumption for a described period. Fasting has been practiced for diverse motives, which incorporates religious observance, detoxing, weight management, and fitness blessings. Fasting can range from quick-time period fasts, together with skipping a meal, to extended fasts that final numerous days. It is essential to phrase that fasting need to be approached with warning and ideally under the steerage of a healthcare professional, particularly for prolonged or greater immoderate fasting regimens.

Different Types of Fasting:

Intermittent Fasting (IF):

Intermittent fasting consists of cycling amongst intervals of consuming and fasting. It does now not prescribe unique materials however focuses on whilst you consume. Common processes embody the sixteen/eight method (rapid for 16 hours and devour interior an eight-hour window) and the 5:2

technique (devour commonly for five days and limit energy on non-consecutive days).

Time-Restricted Eating (TRE):

Time-limited consuming is a form of intermittent fasting wherein you devour all your each day electricity internal a particular time body. For instance, you'll in all likelihood devour pleasant amongst 12 PM and 8 PM, fasting for the final hours.

Alternate-Day Fasting:

Alternate-day fasting consists of alternating between days of ordinary consuming and days of fasting, wherein calorie intake is confined.

Extended Fasting:

Extended fasting typically refers to fasts that final for numerous days, frequently with out a or very minimal caloric consumption. Extended fasts are extra good sized and want to be undertaken with careful making plans and scientific supervision.

Water Fasting:

Water fasting is an extended fasting technique where handiest water is consumed. It can last for severa days and is one of the strictest varieties of fasting.

Juice Fasting:

Juice fasting involves ingesting satisfactory freshly squeezed juices from give up end result and veggies for a unique duration. It offers a few nutrients however restricts sturdy food.

Partial Fasting:

Partial fasting allows the intake of a constrained type of calories, regularly thru precise food or drinks, inside the direction of fasting durations.

The desire of fasting method can rely on person dreams, fitness concerns, and private alternatives. When combining fasting with on foot, it's miles crucial to comply the fasting routine to manual going for walks ordinary performance, restoration, and not unusual properly-being. Consulting a healthcare professional or nutritionist is without a doubt beneficial in advance than starting a fasting and going for walks ordinary, specifically when you have specific fitness situations or dreams.

Combining strolling with fasting can provide numerous blessings that encompass superior energy stages, weight manipulate, and greater suitable staying electricity. Here's a better have a take a look at those blessings:

1. Improved Energy Levels:

Enhanced Fat Utilization: Fasting encourages the body to tap into its fats shops for energy. When you run in a fasted united states of america, your body becomes greater green at burning saved fat, that may offer a sustained and reliable supply of electricity within the path of your run. This is specifically high-quality for longer runs or staying power training.

Stable Blood Sugar Levels: Fasting can assist adjust blood sugar levels. Stable blood sugar prevents the electricity crashes and hunger pangs associated with not unusual or immoderate-carb food. As a prevent result, runners may additionally moreover experience extra normal power tiers all through their runs.

Increased Focus and Mental Clarity: Running whilst fasting can promote highbrow alertness and interest. Some runners record heightened highbrow readability in the end of fasted runs, that could make contributions to superior everyday usual performance and a greater amusing taking walks enjoy.

2. Weight Management:

Enhanced Fat Loss: Fasting paired with on foot can create a calorie deficit, main to weight loss. Running in a fasted us of a can boost up the breakdown of stored fats, making it an powerful approach for the ones aiming to shed extra frame fats.

Appetite Regulation: Fasting may additionally help with urge for meals regulation. Running in a fasted country can reduce post-workout hunger, potentially stopping overeating and supporting weight manage desires.

three. Enhanced Endurance:

Increased Fat Adaptation: Running at the equal time as fasting promotes fat model. Your frame turns into greater green at the usage of fats for gasoline, sparing glycogen (stored carbohydrates) for later use. This is particularly beneficial for staying power athletes, as it is able to amplify the duration of workout earlier than glycogen depletion takes place.

Improved Mitochondrial Function: Fasting also can additionally decorate mitochondrial feature. Mitochondria are the electricity powerhouses of cells, and advanced function can bring about progressed staying strength and better aerobic regular general performance.

Efficient Oxygen Utilization: Some research suggests that fasting can enhance oxygen usage, essential to higher staying power. This effect can be in particular notable for lengthy-distance runners.

It's important to check that even as combining jogging with fasting offers severa blessings, it may no longer be appropriate for anyone. Individual responses to fasting and exercise can range, and factors like popular fitness, training goals, and precise dietary desires need to be taken into consideration. It's encouraged to are searching for for advice from a healthcare professional or a nutritionist earlier than implementing fasting and jogging as a ordinary a part of your health habitual, in particular when you have underlying health conditions or unique everyday performance targets.

Chapter 20: Preparing For Your Run

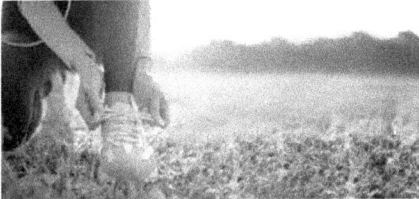

Proper steerage is important on the equal time as combining strolling with fasting to make sure a safe, effective, and interesting workout. This consists of concerns for clothing, shoes, and hydration. Here's why every issue is vital:

1. Clothing:

Comfort: Wearing comfortable garb is critical for a successful run. Opt for moisture-wicking fabrics that assist keep sweat a protracted way from your pores and skin, stopping chafing and ache. Ill-fitting or restrictive clothing can preclude your normal performance and make the run a lot less fun.

Weather Adaptation: Dress consistent with the climate situations. In cold weather, layering is critical to preserve warm. In warm weather, select light-weight and breathable substances to live cool. Being very well dressed for the weather can prevent pain and overheating.

Visibility: If you would really like to run in low-moderate situations or at night time, put on reflective or vibrant-coloured clothing to decorate your visibility to drivers and excellent runners. Safety want to continually be a task.

2. Footwear:

Proper Running Shoes: Wearing suitable jogging footwear that healthful well is paramount. Running shoes provide the important cushioning, guide, and protection to lessen the threat of injuries and discomfort. Visit a specialised walking keep to have your gait analyzed and discover the proper pair of shoes on your running style.

Consider Your Terrain: Depending on in which you intend to run (e.G., on roads, trails, or tracks), you can need distinct types of going for walks footwear. Trail running footwear, as an instance, provide greater traction and stability for off-road runs.

three. Hydration:

Pre-Hydration: Fasting and running can boom the hazard of dehydration. Before your run, make sure you are correctly hydrated by way of way of ingesting water. However, be careful now not to eat immoderate portions of liquid truly in advance than your run to avoid pain.

Electrolyte Balance: Extended fasts can bring about electrolyte imbalances. Consider eating an electrolyte drink or a balanced meal after your run to top off electrolytes misplaced thru sweat.

Hydration During the Run: For longer runs, supply a water bottle or put on a hydration vest to stay hydrated at some point of your run. Plan your water intake to wholesome the depth and length of your run. Some runners pick out to mix water with electrolyte answers for high-quality hydration.

Proper guidance ensures that your fasting and walking revel in is safe and fun. By addressing clothing, footwear, and hydration dreams, you lessen the risk of pain, injuries, and health problems. Remember to evolve your arrangements based genuinely for your specific running dreams and the conditions wherein you may be strolling, whether or not or now not or now not it is a quick morning jog or an extended-distance direction run.

Planning running routes and scheduling runs successfully is critical to maintaining a steady and a laugh walking ordinary. Here's some steering that will help you plan your routes and optimize your walking time table:

Planning Running Routes:

Know Your Goals: Consider your running desires. Are you strolling for health, weight loss, or education for a race? The cause of your run can have an effect on the form of course you pick.

Explore Local Routes: Start through exploring strolling routes for your community region. Check on line maps, strolling apps, or ask exceptional nearby runners for their desired routes. Joining a close-by strolling institution also can provide direction tips.

Safety First: Prioritize safety when making plans routes. Choose well-lit, populated areas, and avoid poorly maintained or secluded routes, specifically in case you run by myself. Inform someone about your jogging plans, and go through in thoughts sporting identification and a phone.

Variety is Key: Incorporate range into your routes to save you boredom and overuse injuries. Alternate among road and route on foot, pick out hilly and flat routes, and find out one-of-a-type neighborhoods or parks.

Consider Terrain: Be aware of the terrain. Some routes also can have steep hills, while others are flat and rapid. Adjust your direction desire to healthful your schooling goals.

Measure Distance: Use walking apps, GPS watches, or on-line system to diploma the space of your routes. This allows you track your progress and set unique goals.

Hydration and Facilities: Plan routes that have water fountains, restrooms, or locations to top off water bottles, particularly for longer runs.

Scheduling Runs Effectively:

Set a Weekly Schedule: Establish a normal weekly time desk to your runs. Plan your runs at times that art work superb for your every day normal. Morning runs can energize you for the day, on the equal time as night runs will will let you unwind.

Include Rest Days: Don't neglect to time desk rest days into your regular. Rest is crucial for recuperation and damage prevention. A regular time table can also embody 3 to 4 strolling days and to three relaxation or glide-training days consistent with week.

Balance Intensity: Vary the depth of your runs. Incorporate easy runs, pace runs, and lengthy runs into your agenda to aim particular additives of health.

Progressive Overload: Gradually growth the space or depth of your runs. Avoid massive jumps in mileage or tempo to lessen the threat of overuse injuries.

Recovery: Plan recuperation weeks in that you reduce the extent and intensity of your runs to allow your frame to get better and adapt. Recovery durations are specially important in some unspecified time in the destiny of education cycles.

Listen to Your Body: Be flexible together with your agenda. If you revel in fatigued, modify your education plan. Avoid pushing thru ache or excessive fatigue, as this may cause accidents.

Record Your Runs: Keep a taking walks log to tune your improvement, which consist of distance, pace, and the way you felt at some stage in every run. This information let you make changes for your time desk and education.

Goal Races: If you are schooling for a specific race, build your agenda across the race date. Include taper weeks number one as a whole lot because the event to allow your body to relaxation and get higher.

www.ingramcontent.com/pod-product-compliance
Lightning Source LLC
Chambersburg PA
CBHW051728020426
42333CB00014B/1205